*Bill Borcherdt, ASCW, BCD*

# Making Families Work and What To Do When They Don't:
## Thirty Guides for Imperfect Parents of Imperfect Children

*Pre-publication
REVIEWS,
COMMENTARIES,
EVALUATIONS . . .*

"**B**ill Borcherdt, who has written several valuable books applying the principles of Rational Emotive Behavior Therapy to people with emotional problems, briefly and yet comprehensively applies them to a number of important family and parenting problems.

He explores many irrational beliefs of family living and gives clear details of sensible alternatives. He notably sides with both parents and children and consistently advocates the REBT suggestion of firm kindness. His chapters on 'Communicating Better and Getting Along Worse,' on 'Fifteen Unmannerly Actions That Represent Responsible Parenting,' and 'Wiles of My Own Parenting to Date' are particularly helpful. Readers who carefully consider this book can learn how to deal effectively with their family's emotional and behavioral problems—and their own!"

**Albert Ellis, PhD**
*President, Institute for Rational-Emotive Therapy, New York;
Author,* A New Guide to Rational Living

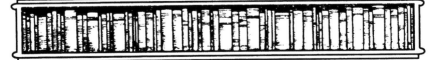

"**A**nother great book from Bill Borcherdt. He provides a lot of sensible advice in easily digestible form. Read this book and make your family work."

**Windy Dryden, PhD**
*Professor of Counseling,*
*Psychology Department,*
*Goldsmiths University of London*

"**M**aking Families Work and What To Do When They Don't* is organized into 30 stimulating chapters that cover a broad range of concerns experienced by anyone who is a parent. Clearly and concisely written chapters hold the reader's attention with interesting and often humorous examples of parent/child problem situations and a range of practical strategies for managing. The book is an authentic presentation of principles and techniques of Rational Emotive Behavior Therapy applied to problems experienced by parents with their children/adolescents. This is pure REBT at its best. The chapter 'Facing and Accepting Ingratitude' provides details on what to realistically expect from children/adolescents. 'Never Deprive Your Child of the Right to Go Without' explains why many parents find it very difficult to limit their child's resources. A must for all parents is 'When Children Double Bind Parents.' This chapter is full of examples and flexible ideas for use in these very difficult situations. 'What the Behavior Modifiers Fail to Tell You' examines the gaps between theory and outcome for behavior modification approaches that do not include intermediate cognitive variable in their design."

**Clayton T. Shorkey, PhD**
*Cullen Trust Centennial Professor*
*of Alcohol Study and Education,*
*University of Texas School of Social*
*Work, Austin, Texas*

"**A**nother book about families? Is it possible to say something original and meaty that we haven't been exposed to before? I didn't think so until I was told that Bill Borcherdt had written a book on the subject. Knowing his style and thoroughness, I knew he would do just that: see the problems of families from many angles and shades, and open our eyes to the reason why some things work in families and others don't.

Take Chapter 3 for example. It is one of 30 chapters, each dealing with a separate issue among families. He titles Chapter 3 'The Role Model Fallacy: De-Sacredizing the Copycat Philosophy.' Contrary to popular belief, Bill does not think much of role modeling and gives us twelve–count them–refutations as to precisely what is wrong with encouraging kids to worship role models. This is neat, surprising, and gripping because one never gets this slant from most authors who follow the crowd and give us the usual advice we've heard over and over.

You obviously can't agree with everything an author offers. Fair enough. But if you're stimulated, challenged, and made a bit curious, then you've gotten a lot more from a book than one usually gets from self-help books.

I've always believed a book isn't worth reading if it doesn't give you new ideas. Rest assured, Bill Borcherdt's 30 chapters will more than meet your need to have some fresh ideas."

**Paul Hauck, PhD**
*Clinical Psychologist,*
*Rock Island, Illinois*

"**B**ill Borcherdt has done it again. He has produced another excellent readable self-help book, this time for parents. *Making Families Work* . . . identifies most of the traps and pitfalls that parents like myself stumble into. Bill identifies most of the myths, faulty professional advice, cultural expectations, and irrational thinking that result in parents' emotional disturbance that leads to ineffectual childrearing. This book offers alternative rational beliefs about parenting, children, and ourselves that could replace our faulty thinking about parenting. Also, it provides good common sense practical guidelines on what to do as a parent. Although children do not come with any type of owner's manual, Bill Borcherdt's book could be the closest thing to help all parents through their children's life. It will help one be a more effective parent–from infancy through adolescence."

**Raymond DiGiuseppe, PhD**
*Professor of Psychology,*
*St. John's University;*
*Director of Professional Education,*
*Institute for Rational-Emotive Therapy*

The Haworth Press, Inc.

# Making Families Work and What To Do When They Don't

## *Thirty Guides for Imperfect Parents of Imperfect Children*

# HAWORTH Marriage & the Family
## Terry S. Trepper, PhD
## Senior Editor

*Christiantown, USA* by Richard Stellway

*Marriage and Family Therapy: A Sociocognitive Approach* by Nathan Hurvitz and Roger A. Straus

*Culture and Family: Problems and Therapy* by Wen-Shing Tseng and Jing Hsu

*Adolescents and Their Families: An Introduction to Assessment and Intervention* by Mark Worden

*Parents Whose Parents Were Divorced* by R. Thomas Berner

*The Effect of Children on Parents* by Anne-Marie Ambert

*Multigenerational Family Therapy* by David S. Freeman

*101 Interventions in Family Therapy* edited by Thorana S. Nelson and Terry S. Trepper

*Therapy with Treatment Resistant Families: A Consultation-Crisis Intervention Model* by William George McCown, Judith Johnson, and Associates

*The Death of Intimacy: Barriers to Meaningful Interpersonal Relationships* by Philip M. Brown

*Developing Healthy Stepfamilies: Twenty Families Tell Their Stories* by Patricia Kelley

*Propagations: Thirty Years of Influence from the Mental Research Institute* edited by John H. Weakland and Wendel A. Ray

*Structured Exercises for Promoting Family and Group Strengths: A Handbook for Group Leaders, Trainers, Educators, Counselors, and Therapists* edited by Ron McManus and Glen Jennings

*Psychotherapy Abbreviation: A Practical Guide* by Gene Pekarik

*Making Families Work and What to Do When They Don't: Thirty Guides for Imperfect Parents of Imperfect Children* by Bill Borcherdt

*Family Therapy of Neurobehavioral Disorders: Integrating Neuropsychology and Family Therapy* by Judith Johnson and William McCown

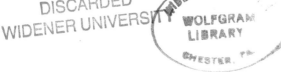

# Making Families Work and What To Do When They Don't

*Thirty Guides
for Imperfect Parents
of Imperfect Children*

Bill Borcherdt, ACSW, BCD

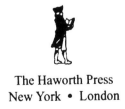

The Haworth Press
New York • London

The Haworth Press, Inc., 10 Alice Street, Binghamton, NY 13904-1580

Cover designed by Donna M. Brooks.

**Library of Congress Cataloging-in-Publication Data**

Borcherdt, Bill.
    Making families work and what to do when they don't : thirty guides for imperfect parents of imperfect children / Bill Borcherdt.
        p.   cm.
    Includes index.
    ISBN 0-7890-0073-3 (alk. paper)
    1. Parenting. 2. Parent and child. 3 Family. I. Title.
HQ755.8.B66  1996
646.7'8-dc 20
                                                                    96-14633
                                                                    CIP

To my friend, teacher and coach, Jerry Hopfensperger, the person who was at the right place at the right time with the right guidance that made a major difference in my life. Without his tutelage I would probably have ended up on the other side of the desk.

# ABOUT THE AUTHOR

**Bill Borcherdt, ACSW, BCD,** is a psychotherapist at Clinical Services of Winnebago County in Neenah, Wisconsin, and is also in private practice in Menasha, Wisconsin. He has 28 years of clinical experience in mental health clinics and 23 years of private practice counseling with individuals, couples, parents, families, and groups who have varying degrees of emotional and relationship problems. He frequently teaches graduate, undergraduate, and continuing education courses for the University of Wisconsin system, and has served as an adjunct faculty member at four colleges and universities. Mr. Borcherdt has over 400 state and national workshop programs to his credit and is well known for his interesting and witty presentations that have practical application to everyday professional and personal life. His first two books, *Think Straight! Feel Great!* and *You Can Control Your Feelings! 24 Guides to Emotional Well-Being* were chosen by Behavioral Science Book Service as featured selections. He is also the author of *Fundamentals of Cognitive-Behavior Therapy: From Both Sides of the Desk* (The Haworth Press, 1996) and *Head Over Heart in Love: 25 Guides to Rational Passion* (forthcoming).

# CONTENTS

# Introduction

This book takes a sometimes unconventional view of parent-child and family matters. These 30 chapter essays contend that the facts of family living do matter–but not to the all-or-nothing degree advocated by social scientists, psychotherapists, and lay people, i.e., you absolutely have to do this, that, or the other thing in parent-child relationships if they are to be functional and healthy. My dad used to say "kids is kids," and I might add, are all different–including those raised in the same environment and governed by similar standards. Families do matter, but not to the degree that they are often portrayed. This text disputes many established insistences that imply family living can't be congenial without certain "musts." It maintains that as the sacredness of family relationships is decreased, pressures are relieved. Abandoning such invisible strait-jackets can then either (a) pave the way for bigger and better things through improved relationships or (b) gracefully admit that relationship improvement may not be in the cards. Although specific behavioral directives on remedies are given, more attention is directed toward becoming less upset when things go wrong–in short, how to make families work, but also what to do when they don't.

The chapters ahead will highlight domestic matters in the form of misunderstandings that interfere with family relationships. They will also show what can be done to better cope with such difficult happenings by family members learning how to overreact less and to accommodate their differences more. Book content places special emphasis on the value of minimizing emotional upsets while maximizing self- and other acceptance prior to attempting practical problem solving. Thus, members will be better able to approach their family unit's transactional problems with increased tolerance and creativity. Contents are based on the unique principles of Rational Emotive Behavior Therapy (REBT) as originated by Albert Ellis, PhD, in 1955. Dr. Ellis is President of the Institute for Rational-Emotive Therapy in New York City. The ideas that he originated examine and dissect the interplay of human thoughts, feelings, and behaviors in unique ways. His ideas help people to unshackle themselves from the interfering emotions of anger, hurt, betrayal, shame, guilt, and worry, so that they can then more creatively choose other more wholesome thoughts, feelings, and behaviors that do more justice to interlocking personal and family goals. A catalogue of books and other resources that reflect REBT and rational living principles is available from the Institute for Rational-Emotive Therapy, 45 East 65th Street, New York, New York 10021.

REBT specializes in using new, creative ways of looking at old problems, making it distinctly different from any other helping model. In its application to family relationships, it cuts off different slices of family interactions and alternative ways to look at them providing enlightenment and emotional relief to family members. REBT maintains that nature, rather than family nurture or lack of same is the birthplace of emotional disturbance. No one, regardless of how they were brought up, is exempt from emotional problems; these problem tendencies are fostered by irrational ideas and controlled by more rational notions. What occurs in families at point "A" (adversity or activating event), i.e., one member harshly criticizing another, doesn't cause "C" (emotional consequences or feelings), i.e., anger, hurt, or betrayal. Rather, it is what the accused member concludes at "B" (beliefs) that either regulates the emotional response or escalates it. For example, "I wish my fellow family member would not criticize me"; an idea that will curtail the negative "C's," or "My family member has no right to criticize and therefore must not"; a belief that will bring on unwanted "C's" listed above. Each chapter will contain rational ideas and messages that can assist members to get along better. When families don't work it's because their human members often do what comes naturally through personalization and overreaction: "What's wrong with me that others in my family treat me so harshly? How awful, horrid, and catastrophic that they do so." Perhaps the best way to influence the family unit is to upset yourself less and accept yourself more, in spite of unsatisfactory experiences within that context.

I can tell I am getting through to my clients when they say "I never looked at it that way before." This is an "ah ha" experience–a recognition reflex revealing themselves in the concept presented. The next step is to plan to put it to good use in home-centered improvement. You as the reader are my client–someone who expects to benefit from my services, ideas, and teachings. Topics incorporated into the 30 chapters include the following rational stipulations and questions. It is hoped that you will have some "ah ha" experiences during your examination of them.

- Do families disturb individual members or do individual members disturb themselves about families?
- Is emotional disturbance rooted in nature or nurture?
- The advantages of making yourself more tolerant of and less emotionally dependent on the family system.
- Uncovering hidden family strengths.
- Illustrating and contrasting to effectively resolve conflicts (how to make things right) from efficient problem solving (how to get yourself less upset and keep your wits about you when things go wrong).
- The value of evaluating a family for problems they *don't* have.
- The human tendency to fictionalize, invent ideas; to actively script themselves rather than passively be scripted by their family.
- Separating practical dependency on family members (especially with children) from emotional dependency (to think that you absolutely require your family's favors and favoritisims to find value in yourself and your existence).
- Avoiding doing the right thing for the wrong esteem-building reasons.
- Showing a more comprehensive concern for your family, not just as a unit who can do things right and succeed, but also who can still accept themselves when things go wrong and fail.
- Why some children will do anything for an M&M, swear by your rewards or swear at them.
- That families reveal character more than shape it.
- That due to humans being accidents waiting to happen, for better or worse it's difficult to stifle human potential.

- Why humans will upset themselves in practically any life circumstance that is less than perfect.
- Why children don't need to be led into temptation. They are quite capable of finding it on their own.
- How silence in families can be golden or yellow.
- Agreeing to disagree—but not too sharply.
- Why changing faulty transactions to constructive ones doesn't eliminate emotional disturbance.
- Uninventing alleged golden rules and reverse golden rules in family living.
- Looking for self-esteem in families as the devil in disguise.
- Why accidents happen in even the best-regulated, functional families.
- A happy family as one who has no cares and a cheerful family as one who has cares but doesn't get depressed about them.
- Rationally discovering wholesome feelings in families rather than irrationally restricting them.
- More accurately getting at the jugular vein of family emotional upsets and disturbances.
- Teaching families comprehensive emotional rust-proofing.
- Why more family relationships are saved by what isn't said than by what is communicated.
- How improving lines of family interactions pacifies individuals without profoundly changing them.
- Defocusing on family-of-origin experiences and refocusing on general human disturbance tendencies by more efficiently dealing with family problems.
- Abolishing human need and worth in families—avoiding the dictating, dependent, and self-measurement traps.
- Family effect and influence as distinct from causing emotional disturbance.
- Creating temporary physical and emotional distance from nonsensical, irrational-acting family members.
- What interactionally goes on in families that contributes to emotional upset as a weak tyrant, compared to what is made to go on in the individual, *by* the individual.
- Families learning how to fish (problem solve) for a lifetime rather than giving them a fish to eat (problem solve) for today.

- Using family relationships as a vehicle for individuals to work on their mental health.
- The biggest mistake a parent can make.
- Not putting the cart before the horse—undamning acceptance of self and other members prior to attempts to problem solve.
- Learning manners from those who have few.
- Overreacting less to different views and accommodating differences more as the preferred gateway to rational family living.
- Earlier influences don't disturb; members disturb themselves about earlier influences.
- Desacredizing and questioning alleged sacred cows of family living.

All of these rational topic areas encourage you to be a perfect nonperfectionist in your role as a family member by understanding and *convincing* yourself of the three core rational ideas of family living:

1. I don't *have to* be the perfect family member.
2. Other family members don't *have to* treat me perfectly well.
3. Family living arrangements do not *have to* be made perfectly easy.

By steadfastedly acknowledging that you are an imperfect family member, in an imperfect family, in the midst of a random, imperfect world—trying to perfect your family role without being perfect, you will be better equipped through rational thought, feeling, and behavior to make your family work. You will be able to recognize what you can realistically, helpfully, and healthfully do and/or not do when your family regretfully doesn't function to its fuller capacity. Chapter 1, "Say It Ain't So: Forty-One Irrational Beliefs of Family Living" leads in integrating some of these new ways of looking at old problems listed in this introduction. As you, the reader become more aware of irrational ideas of family living, you will be better able to abandon these ideas and approach your domestic interpersonal relationships in a more peaceful fashion. Each of the 30 chapters attempts to realign and/or fine-tune a significant idea of parent-child interactions that will pave the way for family members to think for *themselves* and draw their *own* conclusions rather than march to the tune of conventional wisdom. One size doesn't fit all. You are encouraged to choose your own beliefs and methods that will better contribute to your personal and domestic well-being.

# Chapter 1

# Say It Ain't So:
# Forty-One Irrational Beliefs
# of Family Living,
# with Rational Counters and Commentary

Irrational beliefs are those that are not supported by evidence and prevent individual family members from contributing to their families and their own long-term happiness and survival. They defy logic and reason, and consequently defeat the holder's goals and objectives. Irrational ideas are unscientific in that they rely on and reek of unprovable, unverifiable hunches that practically always contain:

   a. A demand in the form of "should," "must," "ought to," "have to," or "got to," i.e., "You, my fellow family member, must realize that one size fits all and therefore you should patronize no other values before mine."
   b. An exaggeration in the form of an "awful," "terrible," "horrible," or "I can't stand it," i.e., "It's awful when a fellow family member betrays what I deem correct, and I can't stand it when they do."
   c. A self and/or other judgment/rating, i.e., "I'm bad when I violate family members' dictates and they're bad when they consider me vile and wicked for disobeying their alleged lawful orders to follow them rather than myself."

Common irrational beliefs of families will be identified, dissected as to whether supportive evidence exists that would establish documented accuracy (DA) and then followed by countering rational beliefs (CRB) that support the idea of rational family living—family interactions that better contribute to individuals' and families' long-range best interests. Last, rational commentary (RC) that is designed to broaden family members' scope of mutual understanding and acceptance will be offered. Comments are designed to encourage members to take a different look at old problems in a less rigid, more flexible, unmechanical, well-thought-out way.

The reference key is:

**IB** = Irrational Belief
**DA** = Documented Accuracy
**CRB** = Countering Rational Beliefs
**RC** = Rational Commentary

**IB #1:** Family members hypnotize other members and cause/create/ are to blame for other members' problems and disturbances.
**DA:** There is no documentation that family members are able to mesmerize other members while wiggling or squirming into their head and gut to transplant a thought or feeling.
**CRB:** Each family member is responsible for his/her own emotions.
**RC:** No one has ever invented a way to give another person a feeling. Family members can please or displease each other enormously. Pleasing conveniences happiness and displeasing conveniences upset, but in the final analysis the individual decides which response he/she is going to make to the stimulus.

**IB #2:** Certain types of family interactions and ways or patterns of relating result in or produce predictable personality and behavioral outcomes in individual members.
**DA:** Because humans will respond differently to similar methods of interaction, there is no proof that personality outcome can be predicted by how others in the family interact with a given family member.
**CRB:** Humans are infinitely variable. One family member's interpersonal cup of tea may be another member's poison.
**RC:** Individual emotional and behavioral problems are not caused by

patterns of interaction, but by interpretation of these interactions. Interpersonal relationships do not cause emotional disturbance; individual beliefs about these relationships do. Family system members do affect or influence each other, but influence is quite different from disturbance.

**IB #3:** Having family problems is shameful and therefore should be disguised rather than admitted and dealt with openly, aboveboard.
**DA:** There is no proof that shame is essential and therefore must be given to the wrongdoer(s) by the wrongdoer(s).
**CRB:** There is no reason under the sun to feel shameful about anything; shame will hinder, not enhance, problem-solving capacities.
**RC:** Shame is an immoral emotion in that immoral refers to hurting a human being–including oneself. It is the human thing to do since a large majority of humans give themselves shameful feelings in the aftermath of public errors–but at the same time it is inhumane because of the immoral argument above.

**IB #4:** Families who have their unique problems should look down upon themselves and be looked down upon by their community as second-class citizens–vile, wicked, rotten, and putrid–rather than unashamedly face and be encouraged to deal with their difficulties as well as they can, within their problem-solving limits.
**DA:** There is no proof that humans are wicked or in any way subhuman.
**CRB:** It would be propitious for families and their members to admit to their problems and disturbances, instead of looking down on themselves for their faults. They would then be able to clear-headedly correct them.
**RC:** The assessment question isn't *if* a family and *each* of its members have emotional and behavioral problems, but *what* they are. Perhaps the most important thing families can learn is that *all humans*, bar none, have emotional problems no matter how they are raised. This permissive, yet realistic idea can prevent self and/or other blame as well as denial. Such provisions of emotional slack encourage a philosophy of admittance therefore promoting problemsolving.

**IB #5:** Family members don't inherit temperamental tendencies and disturbances that they present. Instead they are mainly, if not exclusively, the result of their learning experiences.

**DA:** Individuals raised in the same family, exposed to virtually the same value system, may likely have quite different temperaments, which proves this hypothesis to be false.

**CRB:** Humans are biological creatures first and therefore come into the world with innate temperamental tendencies, which can be regulated with a lot of hard work.

**RC:** Children raised by adoptive parents often take on many of the characteristics of their natural parents—whom they have never met. Custodial parents have frequently reported to me how coincidental it seems that their child is much like the absentee parent who may have never even made a cameo appearance in the child's life. These interesting observations go against conventional wisdom that blindly maintains "children learn what they see." There are so many exceptions to this rule.

**IB #6:** If one or more family member is especially rebellious, stubborn, or otherwise strong-willed, it is because others in the family group have made him/her/them that way.

**DA:** This assumption is impossible to scientifically validate since no one has ever invented a way to determine another's characterological outcome.

**CRB:** Individuals are responsible for themselves, including their decisions to give vent to their nature.

**RC:** It is important to have a sense of humility for what family members can and cannot do to one another. If a family member can be "made" to be oppositional by others in his/her family group, then these same others could also make their fellow homebodies more compliant—in either case an oversight of humility.

**IB #7:** Families should, must, and ought to explain, justify, and apologize for themselves when they have noticeable problems and when family harmony does not measure up to alleged community standards.

**DA:** Where is it written that families are required to act ingratiatingly toward alleged pillars of the community when they expose their inevitable emotional and behavioral deficiencies? In the Holier than-Thou book, that's where.

**CRB:** Pleading forgiveness and justifying problems will not foster self-confidence, self-acceptance, and personal happiness.

**RC:** Public repentance for sins committed may at times have its place, but for the most part it would be more advantageous for families to forego the apologizing and concentrate more on correcting current misdeeds in the future. In short, when in doubt–save your breath and breathe easier.

**IB #8:** Families need to rely on community acceptance, support, and approval before making desired changes.

**DA:** There is a lot of rhetoric and very little substance to the notion that favorable community response to a family name is essential if members of that family are to change the direction of their lives.

**CRB:** It is nice–but not necessary–when community sanctions against a family's members are lifted.

**RC:** For better or for worse, fair or unfair, families develop reputations in a community. The smaller the community, the bigger potential impact the reputation has. Sometimes communities won't change their consensus of opinion about a family, and refuse to give it a second chance. This does not mean that members cannot rise above community scapegoating and do well for themselves.

**IB #9:** At least one–and preferably more than one–family member must have a minimum of one outstanding talent or skill before that family has fulfilled its obligation to the community and be considered to have value.

**DA:** It can't be verified that family members' talents or lack of same are equal to the value of the family.

**CRB:** Talents, skills, and favorable characteristics, traits, and features of family members make them better off but cannot make them better or super humans.

**RC:** Many family members wrongly believe that in order to hold one's "head up high" there must be one or more family members who possess some unique skill or advantage. This often results in families' trying to prove themselves by their advantages, rather than simply enjoying them.

**IB #10:** Past family problems unduly influence, if not determine, how a family presently gets along.

**DA:** There are too many exceptions to the rule to be able to substantiate this notion.

**CRB:** How people think, feel, and conduct themselves in the present not how they have functioned in the past, determines their present degree of accommodation and cooperation.

**RC:** The past doesn't get any better, but it can be learned from by examining mistakes, then spritely correcting them. "Used to be doesn't count anymore" has a ring of democracy, free will, antideterminism, and humanism to it.

**IB #11:** Some families don't have problems, and therefore there is such an animal as one big happy family.

**DA:** Casual acquaintance with practically any family will quickly dispute this faulty idea.

**CRB:** Nothing between two or more humans is ideal, and the problem-free family may be found beyond the pot of gold at the end of the rainbow.

**RC:** Humans are born remarkably fallible and bring their emotional cavities to their family of origin, where they repeatedly give vent to them. Some families may be better at disguising their emotional tumors than others, but ultimately families can run, but not hide, from their happiness deficiencies.

**IB #12:** Families who do not appear to have problems are to be more highly esteemed than those who seem to have difficulty or enough guts to admit they have problems getting along.

**DA:** There is no proof that some families are better than others and therefore should be more highly revered or esteemed.

**CRB:** Good and bad things happen in all families, but families aren't good or bad in an absolute sense—whether or not they have enough gumption to admit their shortcomings.

**RC:** Will Rogers said, "It's great to be great, but it's even better to be human." Families who admit to problems are not subhuman and those that disguise them (and therefore do not seem to have problems) are not superhuman.

**IB #13:** There are golden rules and prerequisites to harmonious family living. A family that prays, plays, and communicates together predictably stays together.
**DA:** There is no proof that when a family does all the right, conventional things, a favorable outcome is guaranteed.
**CRB:** One size doesn't fit all in families and the only golden rule of family living is that there is no golden rule.
**RC:** It is better to have a decent respect for individual differences when considering what family values are best for which family. An insistance upon putting a round-pegged family into a square hole often results in a behavioral backlash.

**IB #14:** Family systems override and govern individuals who therefore can't rise above their faulty family upbringing.
**DA:** There is no accuracy to the belief that individuals are clones and slaves of their upbringing.
**CRB:** Systems don't disturb people; people disturb themselves about systems—and can therefore undisturb themselves in spite of the system.
**RC:** Humans are remarkably resilient. They can bounce back, roll with the punches, go with the flow of, blend in with the wave of the attack in the midst of adversity. If members expect themselves to be more than passive victims of their family circumstances and instead expect themselves to recuperate from, rather than regurgitate, their negative upbringing, they will place fewer recuperative limitations upon themselves.

**IB #15:** Individuals who are looked down upon by their family have to keep suffering until the family begins to view them in a more favorable light.
**DA:** There is no evidence that an individual is required to wait for his family to change, before he can change.
**CRB:** Individuals can change quicker than systems and are capable of rising above them emotionally.
**RC:** The "sacrificial lamb" or the "symptom bearer" of the family need not sacrifice or bear the mark of pain any longer. What a person tells herself about her family relationships is more important than what her relations tell her about herself. Therefore, an individ-

ual can draw self-sufficient conclusions that can overcome an emotional dependence on what is said and done toward her in families.

**IB #16:** If families do not love an individual member and instead scapegoat her, nobody else could possibly love her, and therefore she is emotionally doomed.
**DA:** There is no proof that any one family member necessitates other members' love and that she cannot seek and sometimes find love beyond the boundaries of family living.
**CRB:** Lack of relationship success in one's family of origin does not mean one's world has to come to an end. In fact, one can learn from family neglect/abuse and put those learnings to good use in future relationships.
**RC:** Because a part of one's life doesn't contain doses of love does not mean that such feelings can't be generated in a different context. Some people outside of family may love an individual for the same reason those in one's family do not. This fatalistic belief that one is doomed without emotional family insulation breeds hopelessness and futility.

**IB #17:** A family's negative treatment of an individual results in or causes diminished self feelings in the individual who is selected against.
**DA:** There is no evidence that one person's actions toward another results in transplanting feelings to another.
**CRB:** People will respond differently to the same discrimination, and each person is responsible for his feelings—not what someone else says or does—however harsh that word or deed might be.
**RC:** It's not what happens to people in families that prompts the emotional and behavioral responses in another, but it is more the interpretation of conclusions drawn about the stimulus that causes the response. As George Bernard Shaw said, "Things don't happen to me so much as I happen to them."

**IB #18:** Love conquers all in family living.
**DA:** Love is a great thing, but because all families have problems, including those with an abundance of love, this is a faulty notion.
**CRB:** Love can be comforting and helpful but cannot be depended on to make everything right in a family.

**RC:** If love conquered all in family living, especially in parent-child conflicts, there would be very few parental differences with offspring. Practically all parents love their children—but this often does not cause their children to behave.

**IB #19:** If a family member believes herself to be unloved by other members, the core problem is solved if others in the family group are successfully able to convince that member that they do in fact love her.

**DA:** There is no evidence that replenishing a family member with love will get her past the likely core problem of love dependency.

**CRB:** Even when a person is getting the love she thinks she needs, she is still on a shoestring because she has not yet begun to more fully accept herself.

**RC:** One can run but one can't hide. Fear of being without love can be camoflaged by desperately controlling for it, but in the long run one can't hide from the fact that desperate people don't blend together very well. Changing the unloving interactions will help individual family members to feel better but learning to accept oneself–with *or* without the family's caring will help to foster self-reliance and override family reliance.

**IB #20:** Families change more quickly, effectively, and efficiently than individuals in the family.

**DA:** On the contrary, there is much evidence that individuals in families can change quicker than interactions created by those around them.

**CRB:** By depending more on oneself to change, rather than waiting for the system or context within which one lives to change, movements in the right direction can occur quickly.

**RC:** Because they control the variables within themselves more than those outside themselves, individuals can often make quicker and more helpful headway themselves than waiting for family alignments to change. Some of the preferable ways for an individual to change within a family are to (a) get less upset about negative family happenings, (b) become more tolerant of personal dislikes that exist as part of the family, (c) become more self-reliant about personal happiness rather than depending so much on the family to develop a saner approach to life.

**IB #21:** If a person keeps failing by his family's standards, he will keep failing at most important tasks in life.
**DA:** Because there are so many exceptions to the rule, it cannot be substantiated that an individual's failure to live up to his family's expectations means he will continue to fail in projects and goals outside of his family.
**CRB:** What an individual expects of himself is much more important than his family's expectations, now and in the future.
**RC:** Humans tend to overgeneralize, i.e., if they fail in one or more areas of their life, they are likely to presume that they will continue to fail in all future endeavors. Because humans tend to act the way they see themselves, it is important for them to realize that because they have failed to abide by their family's standards, it does not mean that they have to forfeit their own standards.

**IB #22:** Because family members spend so much time together they should be able to read each others' minds.
**DA:** There is no evidence to document such a family wavelength.
**CRB:** If someone could read minds, he could get rich playing the stock market.
**RC:** Self-pity and resentment is kicked into high gear when insistence that others know what one is thinking or wants occurs. This false notion reflects a lazy-bones philosophy that advocates one "shouldn't have to" lift a finger to get or to ask for what one wants–"other members should know, and if they really loved me, they would."

**IB #23:** Family members should never select or discriminate against one another; rather, they should always see themselves as being in the same boat, sharing the same values.
**DA:** Due to the realities of individual differences it cannot be proven that family members should always be the same peas in the same pod.
**CRB:** Humans naturally select and discriminate against one another, both inside and outside of families.
**RC:** Family members are all different and therefore will not likely

be treated the same. Like tends to attract and accommodate like—both inside and outside of families. A decent respect for individuals, though preferable, is often sadly lacking both inside and outside of family relationships.

**IB #24:** Achieving relative family harmony should be natural and easier than it often is.
**DA:** There is no empirical data to support the notion that relationships between humans must come easy.
**CRB:** Nothing works but working—including working for more harmonious family relationships.
**RC:** Most things worth accomplishing require patience, tolerance, acceptance—and elbow grease—including achieving a relative state of domestic bliss.

**IB #25:** Family members should always be able to find loving, kind, fair, deserving treatment in their unit and when they don't, they should exercise their right to complain, whine, moan, and otherwise feel sorry for themselves.
**DA:** If an individual's goal is to lessen the misery in her life there is no data to support the notion that kind, pleasant, family treatment will be directed toward her upon her command; nor is there evidence that hooting and howling will be of benefit.
**CRB:** There is no proof of a family's sacred duty to provide protection from the storms of life, nor for the idea that flipping one's wig about such disappointing matters is helpful.
**RC:** Much emotional disturbance stems from a flawed philosophy of fairness. Reality is: "You get what you get and not what you want, believe to be fair, or think you deserve." Accepting these not-so-grim truths prevents hurt, self-pity, and resentment.

**IB #26:** The best way to influence other family members is to tell them what you don't like about them.
**DA:** There is no verification for the notion that you catch more flies with vinegar than with honey.
**CRB:** Perhaps the best way to influence family members is to undamningly accept them the way they are.
**RC:** Humans seem to naturally focus on that part of the bottle/person that is empty, and neglect the part that is full. Understanding

and acceptance of others are rare commodities; though they won't perform miracles, they will make it convenient for others to gravitate more toward the sender of these harmonious messages.

**IB #27:** Communication is the ultimate answer to successful family living.
**DA:** Though communication can prove helpful, there is no evidence that it moves mountains as the ultimate answer to family harmony.
**CRB:** Communication can open *or* close doors, depending upon how it is used and received. It cannot be used to solve all problems, all of the time.
**RC:** Surprisingly for most, communication by itself can make family matters worse if not first flanked by tolerance, emotional self-control, and listening skills. After all, what good are communication skills if members are too upset or deficient in listening skills to use them? In families, when members learn to communicate better, their relationships sometimes get worse! Some things are best left unsaid because it might prove shocking for members to finally discover what some others in the group think about them. For instance, "Oh, you've thought this badly about me all this time; how horrible to hear such criticism—you bastard!"

**IB #28:** Because I treat other family members with proper kindness and consideration they should/have to return such courtesy.
**DA:** Nowhere is it written that because one family member is pleasant with another, that the receiver of such favorable tidings is obligated to pay kindness with kindness.
**CRB:** Others do not have to or are not required to do unto me as I do unto them.
**RC:** Family members will sometimes rightly attach themselves in a kindly fashion and then wrongly err in insisting upon, rather than simply preferring, a return attachment. Sometimes others will respond favorably to our best, friendly efforts—and sometimes they won't. With the latter it is better not to escalate disappointment into disaster by demanding a fair trade for your considerate investment.

**IB #29:** Other family members should be just like me, and I have to find a way to make them so when they're not.
**DA:** There is no proof that others must make themselves into a

clone of me or that it is in my and/or the family's best interest that I try to do so.

**CRB:** My family members have free will and can be the way they want to be, not just how I would like them to be. My only choice in the matter is whether I'm going to hassle them for their choices.

**RC:** Often family members try to make others in the unit over, to be more in their image–even though they are not so elated about that image themselves! "Be reasonable–see and do it my way" is often the instructional content.

**IB #30:** There is an invariable right, precise, perfect solution to all individual and collective family problems, and I have to upset myself when I contrarily discover that every family problem doesn't have a perfect solution.

**DA:** It cannot be validated that every family problem has to have a solution, *nor* do I have to try to find something that probably doesn't exist. Furthermore, I do not have to unnerve myself when I come face to face with these grim realities.

**CRB:** Nothing in life is perfect–far from it–including finding perfect solutions to family problems.

**RC:** It takes a long time to find something that doesn't exist. When one tries to find a needle in a haystack that isn't there, one begins to have the experience of the rat in the spinning cage–the frustration of going nowhere fast. It is not a breach of loyalty to say uncle when one realizes that the solution to the family problem is to accept that there is no solution.

**IB #31:** Every family member should be treated virtually the same with similar limitations, advantages, and prerogatives.

**DA:** There exists no data to prove that it is advantageous to treat family members who are different, the same.

**CRB:** It makes little sense to treat them the same when they are all different.

**RC:** One of the best ways to demonstrate a decent respect for individual differences is not to treat everyone the same just because they live under the same roof and have similar gene pools. Some members respond more to praise, encouragement, limit-setting, freedoms, and trust. To consider that fact avoids the "one size fits all" mentality.

**IB #32:** Other family members make me upset, especially when they negatively criticize me.
**DA:** There is no evidence that one family member can give another a feeling.
**CRB:** In families, each person is responsible for his/her own feelings.
**RC:** Especially in families, people are prone to holding others accountable for their upsets. "You made me mad"; "When you act that way you drive me up the wall"; "You're going to be the death of me" are the battle cries of those involved in family blaming. Until family members come to their troublesome family arena with a philosophy of admittance, responsibility for self, i.e., "I trip my own trigger," their chances for relating in a more civilized fashion are remote.

**IB #33:** It is easier to avoid family problems and difficulties than it is to face them.
**DA:** There is no proof that it is easier to avoid family problems than it is to face them nor is there evidence that problems will go away by themselves.
**CRB:** As hard as it may be to face family problems in the short run, in the long run it's harder not to because they will likely continue to fester. It's not easy to take the easy way out.
**RC:** Truth is a convenient, comforting item. An immediate rush of relief is gained when one decides to avoid approaching a difficult problem. If one pushes out of mind the long-range negative consequences of avoidance, while focusing on the comfort of the moment, he/she fails to realize that the pleasure of the moment often leads to pain later on.

**IB #34:** If something seems troublesome and fearsome in a family it has to be dwelled upon, brooded about, intensely focused upon, catastrophized and calamitized about in order to ward off its potential hazards.
**DA:** There is no proof that unduly fretting about family problems helps to make them go away or to cope with them.

**CRB:** A sure way to fail at solving problems is to petrify yourself about the possibility of failing.

**RC:** Magical thinking lies behind the notion that when problems loom, the way to prevent them from blooming is to put them under a microscope and worry about them until your hair stands on end. Such reasoning fails to account for the reality that the more pressure you put on yourself about having a problem, the more you will escalate its existence.

**IB #35:** Getting family members to understand me should be an ultimate, targeted goal if I am to achieve a smidgen of happiness.

**DA:** There exists no evidence that your family understanding you is an ultimate prerequisite for your personal happiness.

**CRB:** It is important to me that my family understands me and it is certainly disappointing when they don't/won't, but it is not all-important or anywhere near sacred.

**RC:** To be understood by those you love and live with is great, but the more of a premium you put on that advantage, the more pressure is felt by all concerned. It is better to understand that it is highly unlikely anyone will ever understand you better than yourself.

**IB #36:** Human beings will never suffer from emotional disturbance as long as they are loved, affirmed, validated, and otherwise sensitively cared for.

**DA:** There is no proof that kind nurturing washes away any individual's problems and disturbances.

**CRB:** Kind nurturing is preferable, but not essential. As such it won't move mountains or perform other miracles.

**RC:** For many people, to be cared for and caressed tenderly is about as good as it is going to get. However, to think of such niceties as necessities puts one at the mercy of such ongoing, caring booster shots. To think that a person is emotionally doomed without such stroking leaves little hope for happiness for those who have not or presently are not able to control for such human warmth.

**IB #37:** Other family members don't have a right to be wrong, different, to act badly (purposefully), not to learn from their bad behavior, nor admit their mistakes that are contrary to their family's ideals. They are to be blamed and condemned for such faults, short-comings, and oversights.

**DA:** There is no evidence that family members cannot exercise their free will in a manner that will prove disruptive for family living.

**CRB:** Though it is better when family members don't rupture their relationships with their kinfolk, due to free will and human limitations they are not required to do what might prove better.

**RC:** The worse family members act, the more limited they obviously are. To expect or demand changes in behavior creates the "double whammy" of their annoyances and becoming disturbed about their irritants. By not trying to make them over, you give them less to rebel against.

**IB #38:** Family relationships are sacred and therefore cannot be taken too seriously.

**DA:** There is no witness to the alleged fact that family matters cannot be made out to be bigger than life–scarcely without trying!

**CRB:** "Everyone suffers when fuel is thrown on volatile family matters. Family concerns are important but it is better to douse, rather than fan, these flames.

**RC:** Making family values sacred increases family strain. Making values important rather than sacred decreases strain while promoting interpersonal gain. When a good thing is made sacred, its value and enjoyment is decreased, and thus stress is increased by exalting something as bigger than life.

**IB #39:** Betraying family values is an unforgiven, unpardonable act, if not a venial sin.

**DA:** There is no evidence that any act can't be forgiven as long as there is a forgiver.

**CRB:** To err is human, to forgive is difficult for most people but certainly possible, especially when attempting to do so without the accompaniment of false pride.

**RC:** Values are important, but the more important they are made to be the more likely that trouble will ensue when values are not adhered to in the family unit. Returning love, honesty, fidelity, appreciation, communication, and other important values and valuable dimensions to family living lubricates family relationships in a friendlier fashion. It would be better, however, to provide without a mind-set that if gone unmet, these would not be forgiven.

**IB #40:** Because they come from the same stock and/or live under the same roof, there will naturally be more similarities than differences between family members.
**DA:** There is no proof that family ties will necessarily breed more similarities than differences between members of the unit.
**CRB:** So far as can be seen, all people are different and infinitely variable, both in and outside of their family unit.
**RC:** It is convenient to assume that people in the same family will be much alike. However, when closely examined it can be seen that people exposed to one another on a regular basis are often quite different in tastes, values, interests, character traits, capabilities, and deficiencies. These realities are often overlooked simply because it is more convenient to assume a selected group of people is alike; thus, one doesn't have to take the time to allow for the possibility of individual differences.

**IB #41:** Labeling families and family members, e.g. "dysfunctional," "scapegoat," "sacrificial lamb," "symptom bearer," "adult child of an alcoholic parent," "codependent," "neglected inner child" somehow helps to better understand them and to help them (when asked to).
**DA:** There is no proof that labeling people helps them to fix problems they seek help for.
**CRB:** Psychobabble fixtures that attach symptoms and labels to people are more likely to do more harm than good because they are vague, mystical concepts that lull one into thinking that such faddish ideas help to better understand their problems and concerns.
**RC:** As problems grow worse, the concepts that claim to understand and resolve them get more weird and magical. Trendy terms such as those listed above are often used to bring a person's attention to problems he never knew he had. They come up sadly lacking the ability to identify (a) how the individual disturbs himself, and (b) what can be done to curtail such unwanted emotions—to say nothing about how (a) and (b) above can set the stage for discovering more healthy, wholesome emotions such as happiness and joy.

There you have it—41 typical false ideas invented by humans about family living. Living a life based on any of these will discourage member's efforts to hang together as a unit, thus making it more likely that they will hang separately. Persistence as a skeptic can pay off in disputing ideas constructed. Not that all constructed ideas are bad; in fact, practically all ideas that humans invent start with what would be desirable, preferable, or wished for by the individual in his/her family context. The facts of that desire are often blown up into a fictionalized demand, i.e., "Because I want certain advantages and benefits for myself and for and with my family—I have to have/need/must have them." Rationally disputing and uninventing these irrational insistances by saying "no" to yourself—that these notions aren't so—you are saying yes to clearheadedness and no to irrational family living.

# Chapter 2

# Examining Your Child's AQ (Appreciation Quotient): Facing and Accepting Ingratitude

Parents often get themselves caught up in a dire need for appreciation from their children. They wrongly assume that if they extend their best efforts on behalf of the child that a fair amount of return appreciation is in order and to be naturally expected. How wrong their pie-in-the-sky assumptions often turn out to be! As a consequence of this brand of emotional dependency they make themselves feel hurt, angry, and pitied. Result: emotionally bleary-eyed parents who approach the caregiving time of their life in a steamrolling, careless, or I-couldn't-care-less manner—in other words, with a high degree of emotionalism and a low degree of reason and logic.

Ripping up this "you get what you give as a parent" fantasy paves the way for a more emotionally self-controlled, realistic, effective approach to parenting. Knowing what to realistically expect regarding your child's appreciativeness of your concerns about his welfare can help cushion the fall when reality begins to kill the dream of your visions of gratitude. To stop deluding yourself is to see more clearly, and to see more clearly conveniences more accuracy in relating to your child. A rule of thumb is that the younger the child, the less appreciative he or she will be. Not uncommonly, once they hit the magic, legal age of 18, they begin to realize that they have lost the leverage they once had and begin to see that in order to get, they are going to be required to give—including some appreciation—lest they risk being on the outside looking in! The question becomes, what is a mother and/or father to do until then? Most children eventually come home to roost as young adults, often with a newfound sense of respect, cooperation—and yes, appreciation. The trick is for the parents to not make themselves into appreciation junkies in the meantime, instead accepting and tolerating the unappreciative nature of the child-adolescent beast. The goals of this chapter are:

1. To identify the rhyme and reason behind offspring ingratitude. Not that knowledge automatically phases out problems, but being given a background of educational information can help to unconfuse the negative return on your goodwill investment. Then, with perspective in hand—
2. To discover how to minimize headache and heartache in spite of child-adolescent ungratefulness.

The following explanations account for the majority of child-adolescent ungratefulness:

a. *Too busy trying to find their own navels.* Self-discovery does not have to end as long as one remains above ground. However, self-discovery is more pronounced in the earlier years. There is a first time for everything—and when your child begins to seek identity via devil-may-care tactics, he or she is left with little time, energy, or inclination to acknowledge your many caring efforts on his or her behalf. "You for me and me for me" is the frequent philosophy of the young'un's search for self.
b. *Little practical reason to be appreciative.* The law says youngsters are entitled to the basic three squares, and then some. In fact, the abundance of children's rights can encourage a take-for-granted attitude and a testing of the hand that feeds to provide even more. From expensive clothing, to having access to a car seven days a week, attending camp, or any other number of expensive freebies, children are bombarded with so many benefits that they begin to insist these are their birthright. If you don't believe that these rights to material advantages exist—just ask the younger set and they will quickly tell you! My point is that in a land of plenty it is more common for children to lead with self-centeredness than with gratitude.
c. *Normal strivings for independence.* Children are in a hurry to

be independent and one way to separate themselves from their humble beginnings is to emotionally distance themselves from their parents. They act cool and nonchalant, even to the point of pretending that the gift horse doesn't matter. Instead they hold to the idea that what matters is plenty of advantages, and the plenty more that they expect to come.

d. *Denial of the other side of the coin: dependent leftovers.* Even as children offer much defiant bravo and limp-handed appreciation, they cannot escape the fact that they are dependent on parents for benefits and survival. They may try to cover up this dependent reality with a "who needs you" appearance to their parents, but behind this crusty exterior is a realization that their parents are still picking up the check. To fog this uncomfortable dependency, the child will often find comfort in purposefully withholding appreciation for the parents' efforts and givings.

e. *The physiology behind "how soon they forget."* Due to an outbreak of hormones, it takes approximately 18 years for the mind to catch up with the body. Until then the child has a dickens of a time monitoring hormones to the neglect of tracking parental givings.

f. *Self-centeredness and center-of-the-universism-itis.* Children seem to have an innate capacity to assume that the world was made for them, and are not willing to consider alternative views until reality, down the road a bit, bites and reminds them otherwise. Give and take, rotation and balance, and appreciation are foreign constructs to be considered later on, but not now, please. I'm too wrapped up in myself.

The following suggestions are offered so that child-adolescent ingratitude will not penetrate your skin:

1. *Use the ABC model of parental emotional self-control to take better control of tendencies to overreact to your childrens' ungratefulness.* Albert Ellis, PhD, who originated Rational Emotive Behavior Therapy in 1955, encourages a method of thinking that promotes higher emotional stamina in the face of adversity, including parental disappointments. His simple

problem-solving model allows you to quickly identify and deal with your interfering emotions. It can be developed as follows: Point "A" (activating event, adversity) is the child's unappreciative, oppositional actions. Point "C" is your emotional response to your child's negativism (hurt, anger, self-pity). Don't assume that "A" causes "C"; that because you are upset *about* your child's self-centeredness you are therefore upset *by* it. Instead, realize that between "A" and "C" is "B"–your beliefs, thoughts, and conclusions concerning your child's indifference. It is these ideas that you have about your child's conduct that interferes with your clearheadedness in dealing with it. At this point move forward to "D" (different ways of thinking, dispute, debate) and try to substitute different thoughts that can assist you in obtaining better emotional results at "E" (new effects, feeling less pressured). How to use this type of logic and reason in the better service of your emotions is illustrated in the following example:

"A"–Child acts ungrateful, i.e., clamors that parents have "never done anything for me."

"B"–Parent says to self:

- "My child *must* understand and appreciate at least some of the things I have provided."
- "What an awful, absolute horror that my child does not recognize my efforts. How catastrophic!"
- "I can't stand my child's unwillingness to appreciate me, especially when I ask for so little in return for my efforts."
- "What's wrong with me? What a bad parent and person I must be for not being able to win my child's gratitude."

"C"–Emotions felt as an offshoot of beliefs at "B":

- Hurt
- Anger
- Self-pity
- Self-depreciation

"D"–Different thoughts the parent identifies that contrast to original "B's."

- "Is my child's appreciation really the sacred matter that I make it out to be?"

- "It's not the end of the world. My life can go on without—although preferably with—the appreciation of my child."
- "Granted, it is sad and annoying when my child continually overlooks my efforts on his behalf, but it's hardly tragic or intolerable."
- "It doesn't follow that I am depreciated as a human being as a consequence of my child's disfavor; rather than 'What's wrong with me?' a better question might be, 'What is it about my child that leads to his behavior?'"

"E"–New effects.

| | |
|---|---|
| • Feeling less pressure | All as a consequence |
| • Feeling more self-accepting | of new ways |
| • Expanded emotional slack | of looking at |
| • More permissive with self | an old problem |
| • More clearheadedness | of ingratitude |

2. *Accept yourself.* Put special emphasis on accepting rather than judging yourself in spite of your child's unappreciative outlook.

3. *Use time projection.* Keep the realistic hope that in the long run it's likely that your children, like most children, will begin to be more appreciative of you.

4. *Borrow from other parents' experiences.* Look around at other parents' older children who have outgrown ingratitude. Ask these parents about the progression of change that they have observed in their child.

5. *Adopt a philosophy of enlightened self-interest.* Become involved in many nonparent activities; begin to see yourself as a person who enjoys life in your own right—regardless of the appreciative quotient (AQ) of your child.

6. *Put special focus on emotional self-sufficiency to the neglect of emotional dependency.* Don't make yourself out to be an appreciation lush, absolutely insisting that you NEED your child's appreciation.

7. *Compartmentalize.* Realize that because one part of your life—your child's AQ—is not providing satisfaction, it doesn't mean that the rest of your life has to be up for grabs or down the tubes.

8. *Conduct yourself nondefensively.* When ingratitude slaps you

in the face, don't make yourself answerable to your child by putting yourself on trial by overexplaining yourself. Otherwise your child may have you right where he wants you—over a barrel.

9. *Administer huge sums of enormous detachment.* Be reluctant to respond to your child when he forgets where he hangs his hat. That way you don't encourage his self-centered ill manners.

10. *Last, and in sum.* Realize and convince yourself that a life without your child's gratitude need *not* be a life without happiness—far from it!

Children are quick to drink the water but in a hurry to forget who dug the well. In fact, humans of all ages often let their humble beginnings escape from them rather than learn from them. When you discover that your child is no exception to this rule try not to take it personally. Let some time pass, and in the meantime don't let your child's selfishness preoccupy you. Instead, when your child shows signs of being in a hurry to forget who dug the well, try to be in even more of a hurry to itemize for yourself how you can prevent getting stuck in his self-centeredness. Develop ways to move forward with your own goals and ambitions—whether or not your child appreciates it.

Chapter 3

# The Role Model Fallacy: De-Sacredizing the Copycat Philosophy

An inmate at a federal correctional institution where I consult asked, "With all the government corruption and with so many well-known athletic and entertainment figures getting themselves into trouble, where can a child seek out a good role model to look up to?" I certainly agreed with him that humans from all walks of life are remarkably fallible and that there certainly is a dark side to all humans. This man asked a common question especially posed by youth advocates. Rather than quickly give a standard answer such as, "If they look hard enough there are some available" or, "It is terrible that more decent-acting lawmakers and other celebrities are difficult to find," I decided to hesitate and think further. After a few moment's contemplation I gave an unconventional answer, that as I now reflect on it, makes a lot of sense. My retort was, "I think that someone who complains about not having a good role model is really admitting he can't think for himself and needs somebody to copy and imitate so he can then blame others when he does the wrong thing!"

It is highly fashionable to blame the problems of youth on "poor role models." This other-blaming view immediately puts the rest of the world—especially the parents—on trial. After all, if the cultural message is that having a good role model is the key to keeping a child off drugs and out of jail—and the child ends up in stir—it must be the lack of good parenting role models. An illogical premise (that poor role models cause problematic behavior in children) lends itself to a logical conclusion (that the childs problems are the fault of the faulty role models).

A young child let loose with swear words on the school playground. When the teacher asked, "Johnny, what do those words mean?" Johnny replied, "They mean the car won't start."

Such an illustration may seem to support the idea of role modeling: that children will learn what they see and hear. Consider, however, the often-overlooked reality that children exposed to the same role model will frequently turn out quite differently from one another and from this role model or any other role model they may be consistently exposed to!

This chapter will reconsider the value of seeking and having a good role model, what such emulation can and cannot do, and in the end, show not only that it isn't the answer to everything in child development but also isn't anywhere near all it's cracked up to be as portrayed by human behavior experts. Furthermore, there is the Goody-Two-Shoes backlash that throws a damper on this seemingly all-important role model mandate. Emphasis on positive role modeling frequently backfires in the form of advisorial side affects. In other words, the pressures of providing the child with an ideal role model can result in the creation of less-than-ideal additional problems and disadvantages such as:

1. *Discourages individualism.* Imitating someone else can seem like the easy way out compared to the effort required to think through and establish your own values. The long-range price of letting someone do your bidding may be that you never discover your own well-rounded nature.

2. *Can encourage self-downing in the imitator.* Discovering that the copycat does not have the resource (talent, personality strengths, intelligence, temperament) to measure up to the exhaulted model, be it parent, minister, teacher, athlete, sibling, often is followed by putting oneself down for not being "good enough" to take on the other's talents and traits that one has so admired and tried so hard to emulate. The misery equation, "my deficiencies in imitating my role model's characteristics = my worthlessness," frequently comes alive.

3. *Invites the imperfect parents of their imperfect children to blame themselves.* Yet, the heavy emphasis on the absolute necessity of parents providing a positive role model, lest their children end up behind the emotional and behavioral distur-

bance eight ball, accomplishes just that. If parents are told that their child will end up eating, sleeping, breathing, and behaving just like them and the child over time displays oppositional, problematic behavior patterns, most parents will consider themselves to be responsible for their child's poor decisions. Lacking balanced instruction—not being informed that their child will have problems regardless of the role models they are exposed to—they do what comes naturally: personalize, blame, and depreciate themselves for being an imperfect parent of an imperfect child. Questioning conventional wisdom about the supposed overriding influence of parental role modeling results in countering the parental misery equation: "My deficiencies in getting my child to turn out satisfactory in the eyes of the community = my worthlessness."

4. *Is antimental health in that it gives blind adherence to a concept that obviously has many exceptions.* Many people exposed to everyday "poor" role models turn out "good" and many exposed to "good" models turn out "bad." The universe doesn't run in orderly cycles, as the copycat equation will lead you to believe if you let it. Mental health involves being flexible, permissive, and open-minded. This is opposed to giving blind allegiance to others' standards—ministers, parents, teachers, therapists—all of whom have problems of their own. It would be far wiser and emotionally healthier to dispute the role model allegations by a thorough self-examination that includes the following self-questions and statements:

- "How can it be proven that role modeling is vital to my child's development, especially since there are so many exceptions to their imitative rule?"
- "Why can't my child learn to think more for him/herself rather than blindly and rigidly adhere to my example, or anyone elses', for that matter?"
- "Doesn't my child have free will, and can therefore pick and choose those role models he/she wishes to follow and those he/she wants to discard?"
- "Anything my child believes and models does not have to be kept alive and remain in effect forever."

- "Role-modeling influence, like the rest of the world, seems to run randomly and impartially."
- "How is it that different people will respond differently to the same role model?"
- "What is so great about copying someone else's manner at the expense of independently creating your own?"
- "Why sell yourself short by becoming a clone of someone else? Rather, to thine own self be true."
- "Self-choosing is better than other-choosing."
- "Would it not be better for a person to follow one's own nose, and learn from the consequences of one's choices, even if the knowledge comes from the school of hard knocks, than to blindly play follow the role model leader?"

5. *Skepticism about what and who to believe.* Human beings are biological creatures first and will therefore tend to go in the direction that they are headed. This often-overlooked reality runs counter to the role model theory. Often children will follow their own nose rather than copy someone else's example. They do this simply because it's the natural thing for them to do. Like most humans they have strong tendencies to motivate themselves by immediate convenience—and what is convenient for them is to do what comes naturally rather than to follow someone else's unnatural example. Confusion and doubt often set in when parents bear witness to this natural happening. For instance, with the first child the parents usually see themselves as the primary molder of and model for their child's personality development. The second child very frequently elicits the parental conclusion that he/she has temperamental predispositions that are fixed and have virtually nothing to do with modeling and family environment exposure. Two different children with similar models and values set before them often turn out to be worlds apart in their personalities! What is a parent to believe after having been told by experts that positive role modeling is the ultimate factor and the answer to almost everything by way of childhood development?

6. *Discourages personal creativity.* Expecting others to model

the answers to life detracts from creatively seeking new ways of viewing old problems.

7. *Limits options.* Choosing from examples that significant others present detracts from many others that could be more independently carved.

8. *Sets the stage for betrayal.* The closer one gets to a positive role model, the more tarnished that exalted figure becomes. A hazard of excessive adulation is that inevitably the image will crumble. Due to human fallibility it is dangerous to want to be just like the person you admire. One feels disillusioned, forsaken, and betrayed when the glamorized person falls off the almighty pedestal.

9. *Throws cold water on self-sufficiency.* Depending on others to demonstrate the good life and what is supposedly good for you is a far cry from depending on your own conclusions about how you choose to live.

10. *Fosters gullibility.* P.T. Barnum underestimated when he said that there is a sucker born every minute. Suggesting that children follow someone they desire to be like and imitate them causes children to squelch natural inclinations to carve themselves into individual personalities.

11. *Implies absolutes, dogma, and certainty.* Suggesting a role model be used to emulate values is to suggest that there is one person with one correct set of values to live by rather than more flexibly appreciate individualism.

12. *Suggests an automatic, magical solution to human growth and development.* Strict dedication to role modeling overlooks the fact that people will respond differently to the same circumstances, stimulus, and role model. Therefore, to assume that certain types of positive role modeling are good for all is a fallacy.

Think twice about the individual you would like your child to use as a role model. Better yet, give consideration to the idea that it is a fallacy to believe that a role model for your child is a necessity to begin with. Weigh the side effects of the copycat theory. Ask yourself whether suggesting a role model to your child might do more harm than good. You may be putting yourself on trial by believing that the image you project determines your child's developmental outcome. Encouraging your child to imitate someone else rather than be him/herself may be a handicap to his/her well-roundedness. Recommend that your child make up his/her own mind as to what path he/she chooses to follow. This encourages a child's efforts to be a strong, authentic individual, rather than becoming a weak carbon copy of someone else.

Chapter 4

# Communicating Better and Getting Along Worse: When and Why It's Better for Family Communication to Draw a Blank

Of all the overlooked incongruities of family living one that often goes unnoticed is the mistaken notion that communication between family members is the alpha and omega—the beginning and the end—all important and bigger than life. Tune into the popular self-help talk shows and you will likely hear a mental health professional proclaim communication as being at the core of family harmony. Read practically any of the popular books about improving interpersonal relationships and you will see how people in families allegedly "need to have open communication." It is often true that the closer you come to a goal's ideals, the more tarnished its realities become. The glittering that communication represents is no exception. This chapter begs to differ with the communication experts who idealize the advantageous role of communication in family relationship building. It exposes the dangerous realities of communication without first pursuing tolerance training. It maintains that teaching and promoting good communication in families is only a fraction of the relationship improvement value. It asks and answers the question, "What good are family communication skills if members are (a) too disturbed to use them to begin with and (b) overreact to what they might hear when they don't understand how to listen?"

So, what good is freedom of speech if the parties involved are not trained in the art and science of listening? Communication training without first establishing a tolerance for what might be heard during open discussions can become an "honestly and openly communicate with me but say what I want to hear" deception, causing very negative relationship results. Upon family members revealing "true feelings," the family atmosphere often becomes contaminated with surprise if not shock from the sender and receiver of the message. The sender often is surprised that upon honoring the receiver's request for getting all his cards on the table the receiver folds and angrily leaves when he discovers, "so that is what you have thought of me all along!" The receiver often experiences hurt, shock, dismay, and betrayal when the part of the relationship that is empty no longer goes unannounced.

This encounter could have been prevented by using Rational Emotive Behavior Therapy to not get ahead of the communication process: Agree on applying patience, tolerance, acceptance, and forgiveness prior to the communication process. To prepare yourself for more well-rounded communication connections, adopt the following rational ideas regarding what you might dislike hearing through open exchanges:

- "Others don't have to say only things that I want to hear when I converse with them."
- "Because I would prefer to hear kind words doesn't mean that others must provide them."
- "It is not awful and catastrophic when others do not whisper sweet nothings in my ear."
- "Honesty in communication means: Say what you want to say, not necessarily what I want to hear.'"
- "It is better to expect some surprises when I encourage others to level with me, otherwise I will be more likely to overreact to their (un)kind honesty and discourage it in future discussions."
- "Others are entitled to their opinions, not my opinion of what I would like them to say."
- "Feedback can be negative as well as positive. It is better to accept this from the start, lest I risk needlessly disturbing

myself when I discover the hole in the doughnut as well as the doughnut."

- "It is better for me to hear what others have to say than what I want to hear."
- "Others words do not define me and I do not have to personalize and feel hurt when people are honest enough to tell me how they 'really feel.'"
- "When I and/or others express a desire to communicate more openly, I am not on trial or required to needlessly defend myself against their occasional salty descriptions of me."

The following are examples of family interactions in which the apparent communication solution actually turns into additional problems because tolerance training was neglected.

- Following the first day of kindergarten parents ask their child how he liked his first day of school. He honestly explains that he thought it was for the birds and the worried parents begin to nag him in an effort to get him to like school. The parents obviously expected their child to like his first day of school and intolerantly refused to settle for anything less than a favorable review.
- A couple is encouraged by their marital counselor to "be more open and honest with each other" and to "be sure to tell each other how you really feel about matters of mutual concern." The wife asks the husband how he liked his favorite Italian meal that she had cooked. He truthfully tells her that he thought it tasted like his favorite ingredient was missing. She becomes hurt and angry because he had the gall to say what she didn't want to hear.
- A married couple desires to achieve total honesty. Several years into the marriage one inquires if the other dated anyone else during their courtship period. The partner admits that he/she had an extra love relationship or two prior to marriage and the mate begins to raise holy terror, threatening divorce.
- Family members discuss their degree of communication with each other and agree to "level" with one another more often. A short time into the improved communication project, they

are often heard saying to each other "So this is the way you have thought about me all along." They begin to realize that something is missing in their discussions. They are engaging in many of the right, direct communication subjects but are getting worse conversational results than before their well-intended plan. They fail because their "open communication" requires each to say only what the other wants to hear! Further relationship erosion occurs because the preparatory lessons for increased tolerance for individual differences and negative reviews has not been put into the communication equation: Tolerance plus feedback = efficient communication; feedback without tolerance = relationship deterioration.

- At a family meeting one of the children announces that he doesn't like living at home. The parents make themselves feel offended and take issue with this pronouncement in a way that ignites the strong feelings of all concerned. An emotional free-for-all results with the family disclaiming each other and any future attempt to hold another family meeting.

- At a similar family meeting parent #1 lodges a concern that parent #2 is undermining his/her authority and making it difficult to create a united front—"we're in this together"—in the enforcement of child discipline. Partner #2 strongly believes that he/she has been trying especially hard to do what he/she is accused of not doing! Upon being confronted by partner #1's perception of the opposite, partner #2 enrages him/herself and future attempts at child discipline falter even more. Here again, communication is (rightly) given its important due—but without tolerance training to support it, it crumbles due to the personalization and overreaction that follows individual differences.

- Two teenage sisters agree to provide feedback of observations and conclusions each has about the other's boyfriend. They emphasize the value of getting "a second opinion." The day comes when one begins to find fault with the other's taste in males. The receiver of the contrary views becomes so angry that she refuses to speak to her sister for weeks on end.

Each of these family fracases could have been prevented by realizing:

1. There is a difference between a white lie and a black truth and opting for the white lie can be the salvation of a relationship.
2. It's not always practical to be honest. Because most people don't take the truth in stride, it is better to tiptoe around individual difference rather than meet it head on.
3. The art of being wise is knowing what to overlook rather than to overstate.
4. Silence can be golden because it avoids someone else's allergy to what one might say.
5. When one allows for and accepts another's sensitivities by side-stepping them in communication, one commits a kind, loving act.
6. An individual can stand up for himself and his relationship with family members by unangrily sitting down, *not* discussing the bones you have to pick with them.
7. There is value in applying Dr. Albert Ellis' Rational Emotive Behavior Therapy. By identifying the irrational beliefs (IBs) that one brings to the communication and by countering these with rational beliefs (RBs) of communication as outlined in Table 4.1, one can take the sacredness out of communication and in doing so lessen the pressure of the exchange as well as minimize human tendencies to personalize and exaggerate the significance of what is heard.

## TABLE 4.1

| Irrational Beliefs of Communication (IBs) | Rational Beliefs of Communication (RBs) |
| --- | --- |
| 1. "I absolutely must communicate on a regular basis with my fellow family members and it is negligent on my part when I don't." | "Sometimes it is desirable for me to communicate and sometimes it isn't. Not communicating because I deem it better not to, does not constitute negligence." |
| 2. "What a louse I am for being derelict in my communication duties." | "Communication is not a duty, it is a choice, and I need not denigrate myself for my choices." |

TABLE 4.1 (continued)

| Irrational Beliefs of Communication (IBs) | Rational Beliefs of Communication (RBs) |
|---|---|
| 3. "Total honesty in family matters is the only way to go, and I find it intolerable when honesty is deemed not to be the best policy." | "Nobody is perfect at taking the truth in stride and therefore honesty is frequently not the best policy." |
| 4. "Our family life must include heavy doses of communication or else it will surely deteriorate." | "The more insistent and demanding I make family communication the more pressure I put on all concerned, defeating my original conversational purpose." |
| 5. "My fellow family members must communicate with me according to my standards and if they don't, they are at fault for any and all family problems." | "Some people are more or less talkative than others and it is better if I allow for such individual differences. It is not these differences that are at fault for family problems, but it is my refusal to accept them that gets in the way." |
| 6. "Communication is a family's lifeline and this family needs to communicate!" | "Here again, better that I not make a necessity out of a good thing, which communication can be, or else I will defeat constructive goals." |
| 7. "For a family to be healthy, communication must naturally and easily flow without regard for the effort required to analyze when it would be better to open up and when it might not be. Also, it is not required to understand and tolerate what others in the family have to say." | "Very little between humans is ideal or easy, so why must family living be the one exception to the rule?" |
| 8. "A large majority of the experts say that communication is essential for a family and that it can't get too much of it; they can't all be wrong." | "Who knows what is best about communication, me or the experts? It is better to be selective regarding my communication in my family, and I can't think of anyone who is more qualified to decide when to choose to communicate than I." |

The myth is that communication is the answer to anything that ails a family. The reality is that if communication is not selective, well-thought-out, and applied with an abundance of tolerance, it can upset an already-teetering apple cart. Communication can result in more family problems–if you let it–by compulsively forcing the issue. Open communication is good for some people, some of the time, in reference to certain issues. Sometimes families who learn to communicate better–end up getting along worse. More relationships in families are saved not by what *is* communicated but by what *isn't*. A family that *doesn't* communicate about certain issues is often more likely to stay together. By drawing a blank in communication rather than accidently (or accidently on purpose) shooting live negative commentary, you can frequently encourage the emotional life of those that you care about most.

Chapter 5

# When It's Cruel To Be Kind:
# The Mistake of Linking
# Favorable Regard for Your Child
# to Human Worth

Perhaps the biggest hoax against parents is the suggestion that they, for ulterior motives, heap lavish praise combined with abundant, enthusiastic love, understanding, and approval upon their child. They are frequently told to do this by the experts, so that the child develops more self-esteem. I wish to be very clear that my goal is not to knock the pleasantries listed above, or to suggest that they be viewed as trivial and without value in their own right. Rather, these external props are not valid indicators of human worth. Instructing parents that these external props—approval, praise, love, understanding, and other acts of kindness—help children develop more self-esteem is one of the poorer methods of advice that can be given to parents. Such a rating-game philosophy defeats rather than supports the development of an emotionally healthy child.

To suggest a higher self-regard exists for those children who are the generous recipients of lavish attention is to invite emotional dependency and disturbance. The equation that "my parents', teachers', and others' acts of kindness toward me = me" is not only misleading and fraudulent, but also unkind, if not cruel. To suggest to parents that they offer open favorable regard for their child is fine by itself, but to provide such external indicators for the alleged purpose of garnering personal worth is to strengthen the child's preexisting idea that "I'm nobody unless somebody favorably acknowledges/relates to me." Children, like all humans, are neither good nor bad. They each produce behaviors and have traits that either contribute to or detract from long-range happiness and survival. They are better off with the favorable contributions and worse off with the negative features, but are not better or worse people. Kindness is transformed to cruelty when parents and children are indoctrinated with the false assumption that favorable treatment strengthens worth, regard, or esteem. The two-sided coin of kindness as cruelty exists for the following reasons:

1. *Places the child at the mercy of others' treatment of and behavior toward him.* If a child believes that his value to self is dependent upon others' favorable regard, he remains emotionally beholden to those others who are then free to push his buttons at will. Blind conformity and sickly gratitude rather than independent thought and preferential respect for others are set as goals in an effort to gather ongoing favorable regard from one's social group.

2. *Implies double messages that lead to emotional seasickness.* If you can give high self-regard, worth, or esteem to a child via displays of kindness, then by the same logic when treatment of that child is less than desirable—as it often will be in an imperfect world with imperfectly acting people—the child will emotionally flip-flop back to misery. If praise accounts for feeling good, then criticism by the same token accounts for feeling bad. Because children are exposed to fluctuating treatment patterns by significant others, this "favorable regard for high self-esteem" exchange will often leave the child devoid of emotional well-being.

3. *Implies that when liked for special reasons you are a special person.* Humans are unique, and that quality is nothing to sneeze at, rather something to be appreciated, if not treasured. However, to equate special reasons, i.e., being liked and praised, to being special as a person is an inaccurate view. "Special" implies anointment, and so far as can be proved no one has been anointed.

To view oneself as special often is followed by these invalid demands:

a. Because I'm so special I must always give special performances.
b. Because I'm so special others must treat me special.
c. Because I'm so special the world must provide me with special favors.

Appreciate your uniqueness but uninvent the implication that you're special lest you give yourself a logical conclusion to an illogical premise, i.e., when important others treat me with kindness and consideration I'm special—so therefore I must get others to provide for all my wishes, wants, and desires.

4. *Self-estimations, self-definitions, and self-ratings have no basis in reality and therefore there is much negative emotional fallout from such unrealistic notions.* Gaining others' liking and approval, however pleasant and warm it may be, is not a valid indicator of human worth. Searching for a connection between praise and worth is like groping in the dark for something that isn't there. It takes a long time to find something that doesn't exist, including a unity between others' acclaim and your alleged esteem.

5. *Encourages self-proving.* If the child is led to believe that any personal value he has is in direct proportion to others' affirmations, he will work like a dog in order to prove himself worthy of such validation.

6. *Suggests that you can do something for others that only they can do for themselves.* The idea that your favorable regard for others makes them a more favorable person is hard on all concerned. It's difficult for parents to attempt the impossible mission of transplanting a more valued attitude inside their child's head and a warmer, more contented feeling inside the offspring's gut. It is also difficult for the child in the long run because it encourages complacency that stems from being accustomed to parents' trying to do the child's work for him. To develop a sense of humility as a parent by accepting that there are many things that the parent can't do for the child, i.e., get him to find value to his life, is a significant learning that can result in the parents' being emotionally freer.

7. *Can be deceitful and dishonest.* Often children are praised as a mechanism of control, not because the praise is authentic.

With a child who is more easily reinforced, compliance can sometimes be gained through such affirmation from significant others. However, when praise is used strictly as a means of getting the child to convenience the parent, a climate of deceitfulness is established.

8. *The child remains an emotional pee-wee.* A child's emotional independent growth is stunted by having to go through life seeking others' acclaim to justify her existence. This defensive self-documentation causes a rocky journey through life.

9. *Puts into practice perhaps the most negative mental health effort one can engage in.* Linking one's regard for a child to his value encourages him to pass judgment on himself. To teach a child the value of increasing his supposed self-esteem by literally judging or esteeming himself, patting himself on the back each time he is patted on the back, will also cause him to kick himself in the behind when he doesn't receive outside encouragement.

10. *Camouflages conditional positive regard (CPR) as unconditional positive regard (UPR).* A child may feel hurt because he thinks that no one likes or loves him. His parents then can go out of their way to treat him especially warm and kind, providing him with what is commonly called unconditional positive regard. As a result of his parents' kinder, gentler actions, the child develops what is looked upon as unconditional positive regard for himself. However, closer scrutiny shows that the child's self-regard is really not the result of UPR but of CPR because his high regard for himself is really conditional. It depends upon his parents' and other significant people in his life continuing to indulge and pacify him with their acceptance and approval. His life remains a mercy mission because he still is at the mercy of someone else's view of him.

11. *Springs the self-measurement trap.* Though it has been said many times in many ways in this chapter, self-measurement remains an emotional death trap. If the child is a good person when acclaimed, he qualifies as a bad person when disclaimed by those in his life. Table 5.1 illustrates the self-esteem enhancement. A self-measurement trap follows along

column one that lists dimensions of irrational ideas of parenting that equate kindness with self-worth. Column two offers countering rational ideas. The distinctions between the two columns show the difference between praise and kindness for the wrong, unkind, cruel reasons and for the right, kind, more loving reasons.

TABLE 5.1

| Irrational, False Ideas | Countering, Rational, Sensible Ideas for Acting Kindly |
|---|---|
| 1. "I'll heap near nonstop praise on my child so that he thinks he is a better person." | 1. "I'll periodically, but consistently praise my child because it will likely be a pleasant experience for both of us." |
| 2. "I'll treat my child with ongoing kindness because I must increase his self-esteem." | 2. "Self-esteem is a junk word that encourages my child to judge himself, which will likely lead to giving himself emotional indigestion." |
| 3. "If I don't validate my child enough, she might turn out to be a failure and begin to see herself as a flunky." | 3. "I will validate my child's good behaviors but also realize and accept that I can't give my child a view of self that is emotionally healthy; this is simply one of the many things that I can't do for my child, but that she can only do for herself." |
| 4. "I'll praise my child so that she will comply more and make my life more convenient in these many ways." | 4. "Granted, praising my child may, as an aside, bring about increased behavioral compliance from her, but I will mainly praise her for its own sake. The praise will therefore come across more authentically." |

TABLE 5.1 (continued)

| <u>Irrational, False Ideas</u> | <u>Countering, Rational, Sensible Ideas for Acting Kindly</u> |
|---|---|
| 5. "I can't stand it when my child feels down. I must heap praise upon him so that he stops doing what I view as intolerable for me." | 5. "Although I don't like it when my child feels down, I can tolerate it while accepting the fact that it may be better if he works out his emotions himself rather than me trying to perfume his hurt by offering extravagant praise." |
| 6. "There must be something wrong with me when I can't get love and kindness to conquer what ails my child." | 6. "My child's inability to cope with whatever ails her is a reflection of human limitations, not on me as a parent." |
| 7. "I'll get my child's mind off his problems by bombarding him with kind and gentle treatment." | 7. "I'll be understanding and available to provide advice during times of my child's emotional crisis, but I won't take responsibility for my good works resolving his confusions and conflicts." |
| 8. "The more I praise my child, the more she will think of herself as a better person." | 8. "The more I praise my child, the more she may make herself dependent on it; moderation might be better." |
| 9. "The biggest challenge I have as a parent is to use all the positive acclaim I can muster in order to enhance my child's self regard." | 9. "The biggest challenge I have as a parent is to not pour good things on too quickly while trying to do things for my child that only he can do for himself." |
| 10. "The more good things I say about my child, to my child, the better, more worthwhile person she will become." | 10. "If I focus more on what I like about my child, our relationship will likely be better off, but will not turn either of us into better, more worthwhile, more esteemed humans. It is better to keep this fact in mind lest I give myself an abundance of ego problems about my parenting." |

The commonly held notion that parents' treatment of their children determines the child's value, worth, or esteem is a dangerous myth. First, it implies that some humans are more worthwhile than others, i.e., those children that are afforded kind treatment from their parents. Second, it encourages parents to run scared, often desperately flooding their relationship with their children with kindness. An emotionally healthy parent-child relationship can be built on fear. When parents learn to display kindness in its own right, they are better able to quell the fears behind these impossible questions: How much kindness is enough? and What can I do to instill worth in my child? When all is said and done, it is necessary to determine when kindness becomes cruelty in order to dispel parental misleadings and misgivings, and thus open up greater possibilities for more kindness and less disguised cruelty between parents and children.

# Chapter 6

# Never Deprive a Child
# of the Right To Go Without

Erma Bombeck said, "Take a five-year-old child, outfit him in a five hundred dollar ski outfit, bring him to the edge of the ski lift—and I'll show you a kid who has to go to the bathroom." One of the paradoxes of parenting is that more resources and advantages made available to your child are not necessarily better. It can be difficult for rich parents to be effective parents, and the wealthier, the more difficult being effective can be. However, despite the amount of resources the parents have at their disposal to provide their children, if restraint is exercised parental-child gluttony pitfall can be avoided. Like the child at the edge of the ski lift who lacked appreciation for his expensive garb, many children will take and take—just because items and opportunities are made available. Then they often begin to develop a take-for-granted mentality that says the world owes them all the things that they convince themselves they can't go without.

By withholding goods and services previously rendered, you may not automatically take your childs' pout out of going without. However, you may well make it more convenient for him to cultivate greater personality well roundedness generally and a fuller sense of appreciation specifically. When I was a child my parents couldn't afford to buy me a new pair of tennis shoes each time I needed them. So, when the soles of my shoes wore out from playing basketball most of my waking hours, I would insert a new piece of cardboard each day in the worn-through area so I could extend the life of my shoes. I began to take this astute method of prolonging shoe wear as a source of pride; I would challenge myself to see how long I could make each pair last. Thus, ingenuity and appreciation became an offshoot of my not being deprived of the right to go without!

I have been convinced for many years that it is not what parents do to their children that encourages offensive, oppositional behavior, but rather what they fail to accept they can't do for them that causes difficulties. Overdoing provisions given a child to make life easier can have the effect of making life more difficult in the long run. Eventually the child gets a wake up call and discovers that the world wasn't made for him after all, that factors in the universe are not at arm's length as he was accustomed to in his family. The remaining four parts of this guide will review the reasons behind parents' frequent urgency to save the child from the alleged horrors of going without; the advantages of tightening up the purse strings and being *less* accommodating to the child; a review of illustrations that instruct parents "how to" teach their children a philosophy of deprivation that is in line with the mental health principles of tolerance and acceptance as opposed to demandingness and impatience; and a review of how Rational Emotive Behavior Therapy's ABCs of emotional education can be used to help parents overcome their resistance to putting the squeeze on their child's privileges and requests.

1. Reasons for parental reluctance to limit their child's resources.
   a. *A "We must keep up with the Joneses' " mentality.* A quest to provide items in at least equal amount as other parents, which will have social significance; i.e., if your childs friends have an Apple computer or a jet ski, then your child must have them too. This prevents the child from reaping the benefits of tolerating product or privilege absenteeism.
   b. *Fear of not being loved by one's child.* Heaven forbid if the child withholds or threatens to withhold his love to protest not getting his way. Such fears are often masked by creating a never-ending delivery system, activated upon the childs' request.
   c. *Fear of the child's interpreting your unwillingness to give as meaning that you don't love him anymore*—or that you

never did. This will result in pressing your own button called "fork over."

d. *Guilt.* Combining the idea that you did something dastardly by depriving your child with the notion that you are evil because of that omission creates this special anxiety. At that point the child has you right where he wants you; anxiously trying to do his bidding for him.

e. *The comfort trap.* The simple nervous discomfort that accompanies restricting your child's advantages is often motivation enough to avoid any and all appearances of discontinuing repeated giving.

f. *Shame.* Public disclosure of your withholding ways. This obviously places you in the marked, lower minority of parental spending, and is followed by self-depreciation thus producing this burden of social discomfort.

g. *Self-doubt and personal insecurity.* If you lack confidence as a parent and self-confidence personally you may rush to prove that you are not such a bad parent or worthless person after all. Such self-proving does not have a bottom and consequently the childs' cup never seems full enough although it runneth over by any objective evaluation.

h. *Compensation.* Perceived neglect of duties at one stage of the child's development is often attempted to be made up at a later time; i.e., a father who traveled a lot because of his employment requirements or a mother who worked long hours out of the home when their children were younger may desperately try through financial gifts to make up for not being with their children at an earlier age.

i. *Overcompensation.* Not having fared well in certain achievement areas, i.e., scholastic, athletics, music, may prompt excessive giving designed to assist the child to be everything that the parent wasn't. Such futile attempts to live your life through your child are self-defeating and will accelerate a situation already out of control.

j. *In-law peer group comparison.* This special dimension of imitative response to peer-family group buying habits often reflects a reactivation of sibling rivalry. When it is viewed as a necessity to keep up with anything that other natural and extended family members offer their children, indulgence of the child prevails.

k.  *Human defensiveness.* Humans often act on their strong tendencies to believe that they are on trial, with their social group serving as judge and jury over their actions. Many parenting problems are ego problems that stem from parents judging themselves by either their ability to provide materially for their child or by their perception of what others might think about their giving abilities. Parents attempt to defend themselves by overexplaining, but such apologies never seem to be enough to foster their own acceptance of whatever limitations they have as a provider.

2.  Advantages of not depriving your child of the right to go without. Until an individual has a keen appreciation for the advantages of doing or not doing a given activity, it is unlikely he or she will seriously consider making a move in either direction. Assisting parents to taste the benefits of getting themselves out from underneath the continual giver role can occur by reviewing with them some of the following advantages of not depriving their child of the right to go without:

a.  *Cultivates a keener sense of appreciation in the child.* A basis for comparison for not having, and then having, an advantage tends to make the having experience a more enjoyable one.

b.  *Encourages ingenuity, resourcefulness, and creativity.* When forced to search on their own people may go down a few blind alleys, but often discover how to find their way home. To expect children to make the most of what they have rather than give them more, more, more is to do them a favor.

c.  *Develops tolerance and patience.* Life does not provide a money tree growing out back. For parents to spend as if it existed will result in a rude awakening for the child when reality eventually bites. Emotional stamina and higher frustration tolerance is created by putting the child's request on hold, until the money is there to *consider* spending it on the requested item or privilege. Being forced to wait for some of the desserts of life is one of the best gifts that you can give your child.

d. *Discourages "take for grantedness".* When a blank check is not forthcoming, casualness about receiving paid-in-full benefits is discouraged.

e. *Expands personality well-roundedness.* Being permitted to go without allows the child to experience how most of the people in the world live on any given day. Such a humbling exposure puts one more in sync with one's fellowman.

f. *Fosters compassion.* To go without is to fail to gain an objective. Such misfortune can set the groundwork for learning empathy for those less fortunate, since one has been there oneself.

g. *Plants the seeds of a healthy sense of humility* that can lead to harvesting a well-mannered, give and take, rotation and balance approach to interpersonal relationships.

h. *Can develop motivational capacities.* Realizing that wishes are not going to be handed out on a silver platter can be a real encouragement to go out and begin to earn what one desires.

i. *Dispels arrogance, superiority, and self-righteous tendencies.* Grandiosity involves believing that everything one wants must be gained. Since the universe cannot be owned, one cannot control for all the riches and pleasures of life. Consequently one will be less likely to claim godlike qualities that others who are less endowed could not possess.

j. *Nudges toward a more risk-taking, adventuresome, experimenting approach to life.* If you can have it all, and for free, you have nothing to gain—so why take chances? Taking no chances narrows horizons, making for one dull life. Being required to extend yourself to get what you want counters such lack of stimulation.

k. *Fosters acceptance.* Often helps one discover that earning rewards and advantages brings about a philosophy of undamning acceptance, especially after it is realized that whining and screaming about being required to purchase, rather than be handed, goods and services doesn't help one bit.

l.  *Invites a sense of mastery, competence, and self-reliance in the child.* A philosophy of "I can do or get it myself" rather than "You can do or get it for me" can begin to develop from expecting the child to pull his load by meeting the parent at least half way in goods and services excursions.

m.  *Signals a vote of confidence.* By requiring the child to carry his own weight you express your faith in his ability to represent himself in his endeavors.

3. How to convey a healthier philosophy of going without to your child. Your child will not thank you for the following sage ideas, but these suggestions can make it convenient for your offspring to begin to consider the value of not being able to have everything that he or she wants.

a.  *Say "no" without guilt.* Understand that simply saying "no" to his request is an act of kindness and is good preparation for the stings of the "real world."

b.  *Use response prevention.* Just because your child is having a mouth-watering good time about something he wants doesn't mean you have to make an offer, or even hint that you might make an offer to land the treasure in view.

c.  *Let some time pass.* Your child may hurriedly want an answer from you but this doesn't mean that you have to blurt out a response. Instead, take some time to decide what is best, and then give your disposition. That way, your decision will not be impulsive and you will therefore be better able to stand behind it.

d.  *Point out the distinction between rights and privileges.* You have a moral and legal obligation to provide three squares a day and a roof over his head, but that doesn't mean your child is automatically privileged to have all the frosting on the cake that he wishes. Let him know what he may have for the asking and what privileges he must earn. This can contribute to a healthy sense of appreciation.

e.  *Remind yourself of the advantage of going without for all concerned.* Recalling the benefits of better regulation of your giving habits can be an incentive for appropriately lightening up the purse strings.

f. *Get in the habit of withholding offers.* Don't be too eager to volunteer the goodies that you anticipate your child would like, otherwise you might give the impression that you are especially eager to contribute and your child will conclude that he is doing *you* a favor by taking all that you enthusiastically offer.

g. *Make them earn and wait.* Insisting that they earn at least part of what they are asking for before permission is granted for purchase fosters patience and appreciation.

h. *When fitting, use the child's request to teach the difference between normal and healthy.* "Everybody else has one" is often the battle cry of the peer-group-minded child. Try to show your child (a) that because most people "have one" or engage in a certain activity doesn't necessarily mean it is in the individuals' best interest to indulge; (b) that if you do decide to give your permission to a particular request, this doesn't mean you are doing so simply because a majority of people agree.

i. *Discourage exaggeration.* Politely but firmly point out to your child that it is not an absolute horror that there is not a bottomless money pit.

j. *Spritely explain to your child your position when you refuse his request, and perhaps offer a partial rationale for doing so, but don't tell him off, lecture, or get defensive.* In other words, don't upset yourself about the child's asking and don't go to great pains to explain your reasoning. No matter how completely you do so it will likely not be what the child wants to hear because permission was not granted.

k. *If so, let the child know that his denied request could be given more favorable consideration in the future.* Cultivate hope and encourage future communication by letting the child know that you are glad he is free to make requests and that you want him to continue to do so.

l. *Inform him of your own limitations of money and time.* Show your child that your decision to not grant a request does not mean you are against him but rather reflects constraints of financial and time expenditures.

4. Using Rational Emotive Behavior Therapy's (REBT) ABCs of parental emotional reeducation helps administer to their children appropriate doses of going without. Parents often feel guilt, shame, pity, and/or disapproval anxiety when they begin to consider depriving their children of money, goods, services, or privileges. Unless these choice-blocking emotions are dissolved, there is less likelihood that the parents will adhere to limit-setting decisions. REBT maintains that it is never the "A" (activating event)–in this case a parents' refusal to comply with the child's request–that causes "C" (emotional consequences or feelings)–in this case guilt, shame, pity, and/or disapproval anxiety. Rather, it is the "B" (beliefs, ideas, conclusions, such as those listed below) about "A" that causes "C." Humans largely or mainly create feelings by their thoughts, and by challenging, debating, disputing their thinking at "D" and thereby taking on different thoughts (such as those listed below) they can begin to experience "E," new effects–healthier thoughts, feelings, and behaviors.

Figure 6.1 illustrates REBT's ideas that people largely feel the way they think, and in turn are likely to act the way they feel.

Don't let yourself get caught up in the emotional blackmail that your child may attempt to use to gain your permissions. Instead, focus on the long-range advantages rather than the short-term hassles and discomforts of shutting the door on some of your childs' requests. I remember several incidents when my son was a child that illustrate childhood persistence and the "never give up–try anything" mentality typical of a child:

- Upon not getting his way he announced: "And now to get you mad–I'm going to sit here and be bored."
- On his way to his room, where he had been sent following an incidence of oppositionalism, he made a last-ditch effort to arouse my dander by retorting: "And one more thing, Dad– I'm not your buddy anymore, either."
- After being told that I thought he had watched enough television and to therefore turn it off, he came running up to me, glared at me in the eyes and challenged, "I'll bet your parents let you watch TV as much as you wanted to when you were a

FIGURE 6.1. The ABCs of Parental Reeducation as Applied to Parental Enforcement

| "A" (Activating event) | "B" (Beliefs, thoughts, ideas) | "C" (Emotional consequence, feelings) | "D" (Dispute, debate, different way of thinking) | "E" (New Effects) |
|---|---|---|---|---|
| A son requests of his parent that a purchase or privilege be granted favorable consideration.<br><br>Parent determines that the child's request is too costly or is not in his and/or the family's best interest.<br><br>Parent begins to consider refusing the child's request but at "B" thinks: | 1. "I must not refuse my child's request because:"<br><br>a. "He might think my refusal would mean that I don't love him."<br><br>b. Most of his friends have what he wants and he might be looked down on by them if he isn't given what they have.<br><br>c. "His friends' parents might think that I'm stingy or think badly of me in some other way."<br><br>d. "If I refuse to honor my child's request I would be required to bear the burden of my own anxiety about his deprivation." | Guilt<br>Shame<br>Disapproval anxiety<br>Other pity<br>Discomfort anxiety<br><br>Resulting in the parent pacifying, indulging the child by automatically giving upon request | 1. "There is no documented evidence that says I must not refuse my child's request, but if I do, true:<br><br>a. "He may misinterpret my refusal as meaning I don't love him."<br><br>b. "His friends may look down on him because they have what he isn't allowed to have."<br><br>c. "I may be criticized by his friends' parents for not being the giver that they are."<br><br>d. "I would likely feel some discomfort about allowing him to go without." | a) New, more tolerant and accepting philosophies (such as those listed under "D")<br><br>b) New, more in-one's-best-interest emotions (regret, disappointment) yet feelings of satisfaction and accomplishment from knowing you were true to what you thought was best for all concerned.<br><br>c) New behaviors that have you sometimes selectively grant your child's wishes and other times choose, for your own reasons, not to—but in either case to do so in a flexible, more clear-headed, well-thought-out way. |

61

FIGURE 6.1 (continued)

| "B" (Beliefs, thoughts, ideas) | "D" (Dispute, debate, different way of thinking) | "D" (continued) |
|---|---|---|
| e. "My child might stop loving me if I don't give him what he wants." | e. "My child may choose to despise me in light of my refusing decision." | 4. "As far as being a good parent or a bad person goes, how does it follow that I must rate myself by my decisions, be they good or bad, in reference to the opportunities that I may provide or not provide my child? I make my decisions on behalf of my child, but I am not my decisions!" |
| f. "I have to make up for all the times I have been too busy to relate to him." | f. "I might wrongly conclude that parents are mandated to give practically everything they have to their child." | |
| g. "Parents should give practically everything they have to their child." | 2. "But, none of the above possibilities are as bad or as true as I frequently make them out to be." | |
| 2. "Any and all of the above are awful, terrible, horrible." | 3. "I can deem tolerable all that may befall me when I have enough guts to stick to the guns of my better judgment in not accessing my child to all the advantages that he may insistently proclaim necessary." | |
| 3. "I couldn't stand bearing witness to any of these outcomes." | | |
| 4. "What a bad parent and person I would be given any of these outcomes. I'd stink!" | | |

little boy"—to which I retorted—"That's right . . . but I had good parents." (For once I got the last laugh.)

The Bible states that it is easier for a camel to go through the eye of a needle than for a rich man to enter the kingdom of heaven. It may be easier for a camel to go through the eye of a needle than for rich parents to be good parents—unless they play their cards right by following some of the guidelines in this chapter. Oscar Wilde said, "In this world there are only two tragedies. One is not getting what one wants, and the other is getting it." Your child may believe it a tragedy if he doesn't get everything he desires. Unless you selectively rather than abundantly provide for your child's desires, you may find it harassing if he never stops asking because you have too freely given.

Chapter 7

# The Door Swings Both Ways: When Children Double Bind Their Parents

A large majority of children seem to delight in emotionally box-ing in their parents—setting the double-bind trap by giving the parent two choices but determining ahead of time that neither choice will be sufficient for their satisfaction. When the only two paths offered are A and B, and when both are predetermined blind alleys—what is a parent to do? The "damned if you do" and "damned if you don't" double bind of family living is often explained in terms of the parents' double binding a child. This is often the child that has allegedly been singled out to be held accountable for all the family's problems. After all, if the child is set up so he cannot do anything right, he makes a convenient scapegoat for family troubles. I think that psychologically painting one's child into a corner does not occur as frequently as family therapists would lead us to believe. Double binding happens much more often to parents than to chil-dren. This chapter is an effort to demonstrate that the double-bind door not only swings both ways, but more often swings in the direction of the parent. If parents play their cards right they can avoid letting the door hit them in the behind as they exit. It is hoped that ideas presented will strike a more permissive chord with par-ents while appreciating the mutual influence parents and children have on one another and the similar traps they set for one another. Such a broad-minded perspective will likely discourage parents from overestimating their impact on their child while avoiding one-sided estimations of their important role.

The following parent-child interactions illustrate how children will calculate and scheme to place their parents in the unenviable position of giving a no-win response. Neither of the choices presented to the parents fulfills the childs' wants since both options have faults and are therefore considered to be wrong. The more the parent attempts to fill the child's expectations, the deeper the entrenchment in the double bind becomes, causing the so-called generation gap to widen.

- A fourteen-year-old client stayed out until the wee hours of the morning. When I asked what the motivation was for her practically all-night expedition, she replied: "I wanted to see if my parents loved me enough to get out of bed to come and look for me." They did. When I asked the parents what their daughter's reaction was to their seeking and finally discovering her whereabouts, they informed me that she bluntly stated, "You don't trust me!"
- A client had the extreme misfortune of having his teenage son commit suicide. As Tim reflected on the events prior to his beloveds' self-destruction he recalled, "Whenever I would try to reach out for him he would yell at me to get away and not bother him. Then, when I would abide by his wishes to be left alone he equally would blare at me, accusing me that I didn't love him."
- A twelve-year-old boy complained about his parents' alcoholism and neglectful behavior. After the parents became sober, the boy complained that he could not manipulate them as easily now that they were no longer bleary-eyed.
- A set of parents got an invitation from their child's fourth grade teacher to attend the class play, in which their child had a major role. The child determined that if the parents attended the play, it would be an embarrassing experience to have his parents in the audience. The child also determined that if the parents decided not to attend, that this would signify a lack of interest in his life generally and a deficiency in their love toward him specifically.
- A teenage client of mine demanded spending money from his mother. She agreed to provide some, to which he replied, "I want it from Dad, not from you!"

- A child asks the parent a question and determines ahead of time that if the parent agrees with the child, the parent is treating him like a child by trying to pacify him. However, if the parent gives an unacceptable opinion this proves what the child has believed all along—that the parent "doesn't understand me and never agrees with anything I believe."
- A child told his parents that his friends' parents were suggesting a telephone authorization before he could stay overnight at his friend's house. After making the telephone call providing the overnight permission, the parent is told, "You embarrassed me by asking my friend's parents too many questions about my stay. I know they think that you went overboard on it."
- Children often insist: "Don't remind me to do my chores; you're treating me like a baby." When the parent then does not remind them to do the chores, not only will they often not get done, but the parent will be blamed for the oversight with the child accusing "It's your fault; if you would have reminded me I would have remembered!"
- A child requested that his mother help him pick out his wardrobe for the coming school year. If the parent suggested the child do it on his own, the child would likely complain about the parents' choosing not to help. If the parent did help, when the child inevitably got at least a partial bad review from his peers, the parent was criticized for not having better taste.
- The child requested the opportunity to practice driving the family car with the parent in preparation for his upcoming road test. If the parent didn't have the immediate time to do so the child complained; if the parent took the time, the child might well argue that the parent was overinstructive.

Rather than try to accomplish the impossible by completing both sets of their child's contrary expectations, it would be less frustrating if parents would release themselves from this double bind. Freeing themselves from such an invisible emotional straitjacket entails expecting and accepting gaps in mutual understanding and compatibility. To establish open incompatibility with their parents is a significant task of childhood; to insist that such staged differences not exist creates frustration, hurt, and anger in the parent. This emotionally disturbing pitfall that comes from endlessly and impossibly trying to accommodate the child can be avoided by the following flexible, tolerant, accepting philosophies about what it means to be a parent of a child who is often impossible to please.

- "When my child relays two contradictory expectations, I need not try the impossible task of fulfilling them."
- "My child often seems to delight in setting me up to fall short of his excessive expectations, but this does not mean that I am required to unduly disturb myself about such manipulations."
- "Sure, I influence my child, but it would be better for me to keep in mind that the door swings both ways. My child affects me also."
- "When my child presents me with contrary, unfair expectations, I can take a step back from futily trying to accomplish them, rather than disturbing myself by taking two steps forward in impossibly trying to accomplish them."
- "Better that I relinquish my role as savior to all my childs' requests."
- "When I don't even try to meet my child's fork-tongued, contradictory wishes I can accept the likelihood of being cast in the role of the bad guy by my offspring."
- "In my book, being a parent does not constitute trying to win a popularity contest where the judges are fixed."
- "I need not lead myself into temptation but can instead deliver myself from the evil of trying to always agree with or understand my child's demands."
- "Just because my child casts toward me with impossible choices does not mean that I must go for the bait."
- "I don't have to damn myself for not being able to resolve my child's 'damned if I do' and 'damned if I don't' options."
- "Rather than trying to talk my way out of fulfilling my child's impossible expectations of me, I can instead choose to save my breath and breathe easier."
- "No, that's right I don't understand"; "I definitely don't agree with you"; "It's up to you whether you are going to believe me"–all can be honest words that protect parents from getting themselves caught up in their child's problems and upsets.

However, the child will often insist that these words signify their parents' lack of confidence in and love for them."

- "I am not required to plead my case when my children accuse me of not measuring up in the double-bound manner they demand."
- "If I avoid overexplaining my position to my child, I can avoid being put over a barrel by my child."
- "My children make themselves miserable about not being able to be in two places at once in meeting their contradictory requests, but this does not mean that I have to provide them with company."

There are advantages and disadvantages to both success and failure. In this sense, life is a double bind—so why must parenting be any different? Yet, in the case of parents blindly adhering to children's wishes, an escape clause can be created and enforced. What this means is parents can accept the fact of being "set up" as being part of the territory of emancipation and ingratitude that they are expected to stomach. Don't take is personally when the door swings both ways, and you won't hurt yourself so much each time it swings your way.

# Chapter 8

# Fifteen Unmannerly Actions
# That Represent Responsible Parenting

Whether something is right or wrong, good or bad often is determined by whether you are asking or giving, and by which side of the fence you are standing on. This is true in love, war, or in parenting, which is a mixture of the first two. Acting against your child's fondest wishes and requests is not going to win you any popularity contests with him/her; in fact, your refusals and disagreements are likely to verify to your child what he/she has been suspecting all along—that you are a "bad" parent for your contrary interferences. When confronted with such critical accusation from your child it is important to hold your ground while not putting yourself on trial in the face of your child's negative barbs. Though your child may be the last one to admit it, your "worst" behavior may be in your child's best interests.

Children practically always define the ideal parent as one who agrees with him/her, complies with his/her wishes or in other ways makes life easier for the offspring. Understanding and accepting that it is not necessary to "tickle the ear" of your children to do what you deem correct helps to empower you to more effectively and efficiently cope with parenthood. The main point of this chapter is not that your final decisions as parents will always be correct but that oftentimes acting bad in the eyes of your child can be good because you are doing greater justification to your responsibilities of limit-setting and enforcement. Two of the hardest things for children to accept are:

1. That they can't always, and that it is not necessary for them to, have their own way.

2. That their parents are not perfect and sometimes make bad mistakes in their decisions to do what they deem best for their children.

The following are examples of behavioral "good college tries" by parents that their children will likely conclude are bad, unfair strategies and actions. Supportive self-statements (SSS) that contribute to the parents' emotional well-being follow each illustration. Because the supportive self-statements contain philosophies of tolerance and acceptance, both of themselves as individuals and in their roles as parents, they allow parents to use difficulties in their parental role to facilitate their own mental health.

These supportive self-statements also make it easier for parents to follow through in making difficult decisions on behalf of the child.

1. *Physical and emotional detachment.* Self-removal from the field of battle means the war can't start. Though your child may try to give you holy hell for going against her wishes, if without explanation or excuse, you turn and walk the other way, you diffuse her rampages.

SSS:
- "By removing myself from earshot of my child's criticisms I practice self-control and cut off any temptation to jawbone about the matter of concern."
- "Better detachment than feuding."
- "It is wise for me to document for my child that when she shows disrespect toward me I have virtually no use for her presence."
- "This is a good way to prepare my child for real life. There too, it is likely she will be ignored when he treats those in her social group harshly."
- "Oftentimes, the wisest option to select in responding to my childs' barbs is to not respond."
- "As a parent I can advocate for myself by staying clear of my child's antagonisms."

2. *Not answering an unfair, entrapping question or comment.* Playing deaf when your child insists that you are answerable

to him demonstrates your unwillingness to put yourself on trial in the face of his dominating, controlling expectations. This is illustrated by questions and statements such as: "Why can't I?" "I'll bet your parents let you do that when you were a kid," "What's the matter, too afraid you might say the wrong thing if you answer?" "Give me one good reason why I can't!" "All my friends can go; You're the only parents who are saying no." These inquiries and comments are efforts to provoke you to approach your decision making defensively—first explaining yourself, then overexplaining your logic—and before you know it you have put yourself over a barrel per your child's directives. In such a circumstance, the inmates end up running the penitentiary. Giving your child the silent treatment puts you back in charge of yourself and your emotions. You can then make clearheaded decisions that are more likely to be in the best interests of all concerned.

SSS:
- "I won't be on trial unless I put myself there and I refuse to do that."
- "Silence can be golden and I am going to go for the gold."
- "Silence is harder to refute then jawboning."
- "No matter what I say, it is likely that it won't be what my child wants to hear. It's better to save my breath and breathe easier."
- "Mums the word—and the battle-stopper."
- "Twenty Questions and Detective are two games that I will not play with my child."
- "Answering my childs third-degree questions only encourages further immaturity."

3. *Selective (in)attention.* Tell your child that certain topics are not open for discussion, e.g., using the car more than two nights per week, an extended curfew, an increase in allowance. Then inform him that if they are posed you will not reply to them—but that you are willing to respond to other matters of conversation. The creates a less argumentative family climate.

SSS:
- "It is better if I exercise some control over what I'm willing to negotiate on and what I'm not willing to; otherwise, I spin my wheels in trying to get my points of refusal across."
- "No blank checks on what's open for debate or else I might spend too much energy, or worse yet go bankrupt."
- "As in life, family life has its off-limits signs."
- "Regarding privileges, enough is enough, but according to my child, too much is not yet enough."
- "Drawing a line in the sand in terms of what is open for negotiation and what isn't will save us all wear and tear in the long run."

4. *Going on a vacation or a night out without the children.* Kids often view it as a betrayal when not allowed to tag along on parents' fun times. They are the last to appreciate that parents' good times away from them are good for all concerned, because parents are likely to return in a more pleasant state of mind. When parents sometimes put themselves and their enjoyments first and their children a close second, in spite of children's demands to the contrary, they exercise the right of parental enlightened self-interest.

SSS:
- "Absence can make the heart grow fonder."
- "Self-interest—putting ourselves as parents first and our child a close second—is likely to benefit all of us in the long run."
- "Parents can benefit from time-outs too."
- "As a parent, I don't require permission from my children before I leave the house without them."
- "If I sacrifice myself and my time upon the demands of my child, I will merely encourage myself to resent my child."
- "Where is it written that I don't have a right to enjoy myself apart from being a parent?"

5. *Spending money on yourself rather than on your child.* Demonstrate to your child that because money doesn't grow on trees there will be times when they will be left out of the dispensing process. This can help the child to appreciate the

value of a buck, and also emphasizes the importance of not depriving your child of the right to go without. Appreciation for and pride in what you *do* have is encouraged by not giving your child a blank check to purchase infinite goods and services.

SSS:
- "It will not do irreparable harm to my child to be forced to go without."
- "I am entitled to throw a few pesos my way–with or preferably without feeling guilty."
- "When I abstain from spending my last dime on my child I prevent attempting the impossible–filling up his oftentimes bottomless monetary pit."
- "Entertaining and enjoying myself sometimes costs money and I need not apologize for that."
- "It is better if I call the shots as to where and how the money is spent."
- "By investing money in my own wishes and desires, I can try to teach my child about monetary give and take, rotation and balance."
- "It is pleasant to give of *and* receive from my earnings."

6. *Limiting television viewing.* The idiot box can become a do-nothing way of life–if you let it. It can also become a battle-ground–if you let it. Suggesting to a child that he consider giving up the convenience of chronic television watching is likely to fall on deaf ears. If you want restrictions placed on this passive brand of entertainment, chances are that you will be actively required to do so. An unapologetic statement such as "I want you to find something else to do," guides your child toward a more well-rounded life-style. This limitation is another example of doing something bad today in the eyes of your child that may prove of good benefit to him tomorrow.

SSS:
- "It is better if I encourage my child to see that life is not to be lived sitting in the dugout or in front of the television."

- "A bold declaration that sets limits on this activity won't kill my child, and if he threatens to kill me for making it, so be it."
- "It is better to encourage my child's creativity in structuring his time."
- "I don't need my childs' permission to determine how much television watching goes on in this house."
- "Turning the knob to off can play a hand in turning my child on to more variety in life."

7. *"No" as a blind refusal.* Not giving your child a reason for turning thumbs down on his request will likely go over like a lead balloon; yet, giving your child a reason for your decision is just as likely to produce a negative response. This is because practically always the only response a child is willing to accept to his request is, "permission granted." Any resemblance to these two words will likely be greeted with open arms; any responses on the negative side will likely be greeted with clenched fists! When you sense that no reason would be good enough for refusing the child's request, do not attempt parental justification. This can save you the wear and tear of trying to do the impossible–convincing the child of something he refuses to be convinced of. Therefore no explanation is often better than a laundry list of rationales.

SSS:
- "Little does my child realize that an important ingredient of happiness is being forced to go without."
- "No can be an intended love word. Whether my child takes it that way is up to him."
- "To try to document my reasons in this case will likely prove to be more trouble than it's worth."
- "How many reasons will likely be enough for my child. Too many I say–so better none than some."

8. *Taking away or limiting use of the telephone.* Getting on the horn and staying there seems to be the birthright of all children, especially teenagers. The fact that others in the family might wish to use the telephone to communicate with the outside

world is often overlooked by the babbling child or adolescent. Unless forthrightly told when their telephone conversation time is up, they are likely to overextend their telephone talk time to last the evening. As in a lot of child-adolescent annoying behaviors, it is usually better to confront them sooner rather than later. Thus bad habits will be less entrenched and a build-up of resentment will be less likely to occur.

SSS:
- "My child's talking on the telephone constitutes a privilege, not a right. It is up to me how far that privilege is to be extended."
- "As with a lot of things, telephone usage is better shared than dominated."
- "So if I am designated by my child as the bad guy for forcing relinquishment of telephone usage–what else is new?"
- "If I limit my child's telephone use, opportunity to attend to other responsibilities is made available."
- "I'm not looking to win any popularity contests with my child by establishing telephone time limitations."
- "It is better when I don't make myself dependent upon my child's understanding and liking my limit-setting."

9. *Groundings.* Penalizing your child by forcing her to stay close to home may teach the child the advantages of more obedient behavior in the future, but it ordinarily doesn't win you any medals from her in the short run. Yet, such disciplinary procedures are an important ingredient in shaping your childs' behavior. Keeping the child close to home as a reminder of her misdeeds can more easily be administered behind some of the following no-nonsense, emotionally self-protective declarations.

SSS:
- "It is my responsibility to ensure that there is some hell to pay when my child misbehaves."
- "All through life my child will have a fiddler to pay. For now I'm the designated player."

- "Let my child decide for herself whether she would rather goof off and be grounded or play ball by the house rules and have freer reign."
- "Better that I be the warden now, then she face one later."
- "The disobedience buck stops here!"
- "Homebound may be the cure for contradictory behavior."

10. *Playing detective in monitoring your child's whereabouts.* One of the last things your child wants from you is supervision of his activities and whereabouts. From his standpoint he doesn't want to be treated as a child, which is likely to be in contrast with your goal of sleeping better at night knowing what he is or is not up to. Though unasked to do so, part of your parental responsibility is to track what is going on in your childs' life when he is not around—regardless of how much disapproval of your monitoring is given.

SSS:
- "I sleep better when I know beyond a reasonable doubt the comings and goings of my child's life."
- "A certain amount of detective work is part of the parental role, and whether my child or I like it is beside the point."
- "Better I pursue the checkup process so I have a better idea of what to expect."
- "As a parent I can unapologetically make my own independent observations of what is happening in my child's life. I don't need permission to do so."

11. *Call their bluff.* Children sometimes seem surprised if you convey the message, "OK, if you wish to jump go ahead and do it." I recently spoke with a mother whose daughter had complained about what she viewed as her mother's deficiencies. She told her daughter, "If you think you can find a better mother than me, you are welcome to try." A little confrontation by the parent can often give the child a sneak preview of what reality minus present disadvantages *and* advantages might be like.

SSS:
- "Let them find out for themselves."

- "Maybe it would be good for them to find out what life is like outside of the home."
- "I don't have to hold myself captive to my child's threats."
- "Let them find out whether reality is really as sweet as they picture it to be."
- "Maybe after finding out what a cold, cruel world we live in he will be more appreciative of the comforts of home."
- "I'm not going to reason them out of the image of the ideal world that they haven't been reasoned into."
- "They don't have to love it to not leave it, but that's up to them."

12. *Disregarding the child's complaints that his/her views are discounted.* The institution is better run by the wardens than the inmates. When push comes to shove and there is no room for compromise, someone would do well to take the bull by the horns and make an enforceable decision. Better that this be the warden in the case of the institution and the parent in the home. The parent(s) as a majority rules, and though it is highly preferable that the leader's decision be understood, it is not vitally important that it is.

SSS:
- "I cannot force my show of interest in my child, onto my child."
- "My child's complaints about my alleged disinterest are likely just another benchmark of his efforts to separate himself from me."
- "I'm not going to sell my child a used car he doesn't want nor convince him of something he doesn't want to be convinced of."
- "Although I want my child to understand that I am interested in his opinions, it is not absolutely necessary that he see this or any other good intention on my part."

13. *Setting aside time for studying and expecting the child to use it for that purpose.* Trying to get the child to see that succeeding in school is preceded by the will to prepare can be like trying to fit a round peg into a square hole. Seeing to it that

play does come before work–but only in the dictionary–is usually an idea that is ill-received by your child. Yet enforcing the schoolwork first and play second better furthers the learning process.

SSS:
- "(Home)work before play in gaining real and homelife advantages."
- "My child doesn't have to like what I expect of him academically in order for him to get his nose in his books."
- "I'm not asking that my child succeed at school, but rather to try to prepare to succeed."
- "School without studying is like getting paid without working–unrealistic in both cases."

14. *The parents declare that they are going on a strike against some of the advantages they provide.* Just as labor unions, parents can declare a work stoppage of their own when their child refuses to work according to parental specifications. When the parent finds his back has not been scratched for sometime, he can refuse to scratch the child's back. Declaring a sit-down, hands-off approach to provisions previously provided, i.e., laundry not being done, transportation not being provided, meals not being made, can get the child's attention while conveying the message that there are no more free lunches or blank checks and that in order to get, the child is now being required to give.

SSS:
- "There's little by way of free lunch outside this home and it is better if I make that reality consistent with what my child expects in the home."
- "If my child chooses to not scratch my back, I'll be damned if I'll scratch his."
- "Why would my child comply if there is no penalty for noncompliance?"
- "Perhaps my work stoppage will jolt my child's light bulb enough to go on."

- "A little elbow-grease appreciation from my child would be appreciated by me, and until my child gives some I will back off."
- "I could continue to let myself be taken for granted, but I refuse to do so any longer."

15. *At most, minimally respond to the child's complaints about his dire "needs" for love, approval, attention, and praise not being met.* Little frustrates the child more than when his parents refuse to continue to attempt to fill the bottomless pit of the above alleged necessities. How much attention, praise, and other favorable parental recognition is enough? Often, too much is not enough. Moderation in positive recognition of your child, flanked by ignoring on the one hand and gushing acclaim on the other, is often the desirable medium in addressing the child's beefs about seeming deficiencies in these soft areas. Not bending over backwards to supply the child's interpersonal demands may seem like a cold thing to do but better to err in the direction of moderation than of excess.

SSS:
- "If my child doesn't realize by now that I'm for and not against his best interests, he may never realize it—at least not at this time of his life."
- "I have no cartwheels and handstands when it comes to proving my love and appreciation for my child."
- "The less said to defend myself, the better."
- "Sometimes the best response to a complaint is to not respond—otherwise I may encourage demandingness and immaturity."
- "If I take my child's complaints personally, I'll just be setting up an overkill in the wrong direction."
- "I've already put my best foot forward in my softening behaviors toward my child, and this is as far as I can go on the matter."

The role of a parent contains many paradoxes. Unmannerly conduct in the service of fulfilling parental responsibilities is a prime example of such reversals. Your child is likely to be one of the last to understand your no-nonsense efforts as being in his best interests. Perhaps in the long run your child may realize that your well-intended, firm, unmannerly actions were really the right methods after all.

# Chapter 9

# Minding Less
# When Your Child Doesn't Mind

Most people don't like to be ignored and will often do whatever it takes not to end up living in a relationship vacuum. Literally turning your back and walking away from your child's misbehavior reminds me of William Faulkner's thought, "If I had a choice between feeling pain and feeling nothing, I'd rather feel pain." Having nothing to do with someone who has nothing better to do than to disregard and disrespect your authority allows you added time to enjoy life. Children often don't like to mind their parents and tend to do so even less when they realize that this behavior has a controlling impact on their parent. When parents ignore their child following the child's disrespect, less incentive is provided for the child to continue his or her difficult conduct. When parents act upon the idea that they are not duty bound to get their child to mind, a different mind-set, with a swinging of the balance of power, is created. No longer does the parent make him or herself emotionally dependent, obligated to "get" the child to mind. Consequently, the parent puts him or herself in a better position to be less defensive and explaining, and more free-wheeling and self-accepting in his or her approach to the parenting role.

Not that there aren't exceptions to the rule. You best not ignore when your child attempts to dismantle or to burn down your home. You best not overlook when your child is being verbally and/or physically abusive to someone who can't defend himself or who doesn't have the emotional stamina to walk away. To do so would be foolheardy. There is a place for stern, disciplinary reprimand where you draw a clear line in the sand and inform your unkind-acting child, "no more–or else." However, the everyday annoy-ances of rudeness, impatience, and otherwise troublesome behavior are found in practically every child in large doses. Paying less heed, minding less when your child doesn't mind may be just the tonic to quietly but swiftly put him in his place.

The advantages of parenting with a cold shoulder include:

1. Conveys the reality of no free lunch. Relationships usually work better when they are earned, and parent-child relation-ships are no exception. Demonstrating to your child your readiness to Abruptly–with a capital A–walking away from him when he acts badly toward you highlights this reality.
2. Saves you time and energy. Show your child that you have more important things to do than to bother yourself about his whims.
3. Encourages appreciation. Bowing out and backing away from your child's antagonisms discourages the "take for grantedness" that often results in the child taking advantage of the parents in other ways.
4. Demonstrates that actions speak louder than words and that a picture is worth one thousand of the latter. Decisively cutting your child off by paying no attention to his obnoxious behav-ior shows the child he will get no response from you when he moans and groans about not getting his way.
5. Allows you to stand up for yourself while taking your child's contrary behavior sitting down or walking decisively away from him.
6. Magnifies the fact that you mean business by distancing and protecting yourself from his displeasing actions.
7. Reflects that it can be kind to be cruel. Nowhere else on this planet is your child's aggravating behavior likely to be wel-comed. Your refusal to expose yourself to his prickles kindly demonstrates what he can expect from others when he acts cruelly.
8. Builds up your own tolerance levels. By not arguing the point and instead refusing to fight fire with fire by walking away, you increase your restraint and tolerance abilities. Perhaps

the ultimate goal of being a parent is being able to use the trials and tribulations of that role to work on your own mental health.

9. Uses the element of surprise in a constructive way. After multiple banterings with your child over time, he may feel quite flabbergasted when you give him the silent treatment. This surprising turnabout on your part is a signal that something different in discipline and conflict management may be in the air. This can have a tilting affect that throws the child off balance wondering, "What's next?" Such wonderment can be a factor in lessening your child's antagonistic attitude. This unbalancing of a child can promptly promote a balance of power leaning more in the parents' direction.

10. Invites respect. Demonstrate the emotional stamina necessary to not turn the other cheek, but yet turn away from unkindly conduct. This not only can dissolve the unpleasant deed and critical thought and hostile feeling that created it, but also calls attention to reasons to respect such an individual who has the capacity to exercise emotional restraint rather than remain in the line of fire.

11. Leaves better possibilities that your child will overreact less now and in the future. Observing the advantages of the parents' walking away from trouble with the child left holding the bag can be a source of enlightenment for the child that may discourage him from trying to get the parents goat in the future.

12. Giving your child the cold shoulder can have a thawing out effect. This paradox supports the idea that by taking two steps back and no steps forward you can forestall conflicts and arguments between parents and children. By not playing into your child's oppositionalism you nip in the bud what otherwise might be differences that make it difficult to lead a more peaceful coexistence.

In Table 9.1, I will review some irrational beliefs of children that prompt them to mind less, followed by rational ideas parents can use that allow them to mind less in the face of their child's seeming mindless conduct.

TABLE 9.1

| Irrational Beliefs of Offspring That Result in Testing and Exceeding Parental Limits | Rational Ideas of Parents That Allow Them to Ignore Their Child's Complaints, Retorts, and Misconduct |
|---|---|
| • "I don't have to mind my parents—and I'll prove it." | • "This too will pass." |
| • "I have the right to run my own life and nobody better tell me any different." | • "Take a step back—not two steps forward." |
| • "They can't tell me what to do." | • "Give it the limp hand rather than the heavy hand in certain situations." |
| • "They better not stand in my way." | • "Sometimes the best response is no response." |
| • "I'll make my own decisions; it's my life not theirs." | • "The art of being wise can be what to overlook." |
| • "I didn't ask to be born and so I don't have to ask them what I can and cannot do." | • "Silence can be golden." |
| • "They better stay out of my way." | • "If my child wants a response from me he will be required to be more civilized." |
| • "It's a free country and I can say and do whatever I want to." | • "I'm not going to buy into my child's complaints because the price is too high—and that is only at the suggested retail value!" |
| • "I'm old enough to know what is best for me." | • "Overlook, don't stare or even look." |
| • "Other kids can do it and so I should be able to." | • "Don't add fuel to the fire." |
| • "I should be able to decide what my own privileges are." | • "Don't make a temporary problem into a more permanent one." |
| | • "Back yourself up by backing off." |
| | • "My child's conversation with me can be purchased by fair play." |

Try to be of better cheer by using your mind constructively. Encourage your child to do the same—more by what you *don't* say and do, than by what you do say and do. Coping better with your child's critical, complaining antics is not totally a question of mind over matter. However, by understanding and accepting the humility required to better determine what you can and can't do for your child, giving up the impossible dream of creating your child's happiness along with such a fine-tuned determination, you are not exactly giving off the message that "I don't mind and you don't matter," but rather "I will be less concerned to think your negative conduct matters when it comes to matters of importance in my life." Such an attitude of emotional detachment may be one of the ingredients that allows you to clearheadedly pave the way for sturdier, more constructive attachments in the future—once your child learns that you have learned what *not* to do.

# Chapter 10

# The Merits of Extracting Emotional Dependency from the Parental Equation

"I love you very much dear, but I don't need you." This position statement from a wise mother of a teenage daughter that I counseled often still rings in my ears when I begin to problem solve with a parent who approaches the description of his/her concerns with an obvious sense of fear, urgency, and desperation. It would prevent emotional upset and be more practical if my current client could quickly jump ahead to the self-reliant view of my more learned client. I try to get parent clients to the point of emotional un-dependence, and when successful they often are able to either constructively resolve the original presenting problem, or to gracefully accept the inability to do so. Emotionally dependent parents are fearful because of what they think their child's ill-advised behaviors say about them as parents. A sure way to fail is to make yourself deathly afraid of failing; fearful parents don't solve problems very well. Undoing emotional dependency so that the parent isn't afraid of the child's problematic behavior stimulates more clearheadedness and creativity in approaching inevitable child-adolescent problems.

Parents who present concerns about their child's behavior often present themselves feeling angry and hostile toward their child, describing chronic argumentation between the two. However, behind practically every embittered parent is a frightened parent—frightened that until there is a turnaround in the child's bad behavior, he/she as a parent will remain bad, vile, wicked. This condemning self-view elicits the idea that "I absolutely have to find solutions to my child's problems and disturbances. If I don't I have to judge my parenting and myself as bad." In this sense most parental problems are ego problems since a majority of parents make themselves emotionally dependent on raising an emotionally healthy child. They wrongly believe that "Not only do I engage in my parenting, but I am my parenting." The logical outgrowth of such a faulty assumption is "Because I define myself by my parenting if my child does not shape up, then I as a human being will have to ship out." An emotional dependency is an insistence that is voiced in the form of a "have to," "should," "must," "ought to," "have got to" with the implication that "if I don't do what is necessary to do, I'm no good!" Subtracting and extracting the perfectionistic requirements from parental efforts to achieve can be emotionally liberating, leading to clearer problem solving.

This chapter will build a case for parental emotional self-control and self-acceptance rather than emotional upset and self-blame. It will identify those alleged "essentials" (the "have to's," "shoulds," "ought to's," "got to's," "supposed to's") of parenting along with advocating the advisability of countering such flawed viewpoints. Dimensions of emotional dependency in parent-child relationships, parental self-statements that cause these dependent leanings, and countering self-statements that help to resolve and dissolve clinging inclinations include:

1. *Need for child compliance.* When parents convince themselves that their child doesn't "have to" comply with their wishes, much pressure is taken off all concerned. With pressure now under wraps, bigger and better things are more likely to happen on the home front. Perhaps the two biggest stress producing words in the English language are "have to." Minimizing such demanding self-talk can shed more favorable emotional light on family interactions. Rigid statements that demand what can't be controlled–a child's compliance with house and societal rules include:
   - "My child must obey and I can't stand it when he doesn't."
   - "She has to do what she is told, and what a catastrophe that she doesn't."
   - "She ought to cooperate more and it's more than mortifying when she doesn't."

- "He should listen to me more and it's awful when he doesn't."
- "She has got to shape up. How horrible that she has not as yet done so."
- "He needs to understand the limits and I am to blame for not getting him to that point of understanding."
- "My child's indecent behavior is a reflection on me. Therefore, in order to live with myself I have to see to it that her conduct improves."
- "I must come up with solutions to my child's bad problems—or else I'm bad."
- "Until I pull tactics out of my hat to guarantee my child's obedience I must shame myself for not righting my child's wrong."
- "Others will judge me by my parenting and so should I."

More flexible self-comments that accept noncompliance that can't be changed are:

- "I do not have to find solutions to my child's problems and upsets."
- "Granted, I have a moral obligation to try to raise my child well, but such good-willed efforts are a far cry from perfect."
- "Granted, others will likely judge me by my parenting, but it's certainly not mandatory that I foolishly do the same."
- "My child has free will and can live with the consequences of his noncompliance—just like anyone else."
- "As annoying as I may find my child's oppositional behavior, it is still within the bounds of life, not bigger than life. Therefore, it is perhaps not well within but certainly within my tolerance limitations."
- "There is a long-range consequence for every disobedient, noncompliant decision that my child makes. That reality is likely to cause her to change than all my nagging and insisting put together."
- "Life is for lessons. It is better if I stay out of the way as my child learns lessons from reality talking back."

- "The future will likely come home to roost; there is a piper my child will likely be required to pay as his disobedience lengthens. Perhaps then he will learn what my futile preachings have been all about."

2. *Need for approval.* As part of a more general pattern of disapproval anxiety, parents often raise emotional havoc within themselves and in their relationship with their child. Requirements for their child's liking and approval can be seen in the following self-statements:
   - "I need my child's approval and how bitter being a parent is without it."
   - "When my child forsakes me, my life is not as complete as it should be."
   - "There must be something wrong with me if I can't even get my own offspring to support my values."
   - "When my relationship with my child is bad, life is bad."
   - "After all the extra effort I have invested to provide my child with opportunities galore, I have a right to insist that he favorably recognize me."

Ideas that attack approval-seeking tendencies en route to establishing more parental bargaining power are:
   - "Gaining and maintaining my child's approval is nice but not necessary."
   - "When I project a dire need for my child's approval I lose authority and leverage in accomplishing my job as a parent."
   - "Preferring my child's approval, yes! Having to have it, no!"
   - "Caving in to my child's disapproval causes me to wonder who's running the institution—the warden or the inmates."
   - "Because I would like my child's approval doesn't mean that I must grovel to get it."

3. *Need for communication and consensus.* Parents often place two demands on their communication with their children: (1) "We absolutely must communicate" and (2) "You must say what I think is correct rather than what you think is correct and what I don't want to hear." Regarding the latter point, relation-

ships aren't built so much upon communication per se, but on being more tolerant and accepting of the controversy you encounter in conversation. When the parent makes him or herself emotionally dependent upon parent-child communication, the child will use this to control the parent by communiting less. It is healthy to convey the impression that you want to communicate with your child and to make yourself available to do so. It is unhealthy, however, to relay the idea that your relationship life with and your emotional life about your child depends on it. The more you try to force the issue of communication down your child's throat, the more you set yourself up to be emotionally devoured by your offspring.

Parental self-instructions that tip the hand of parental demands for communication include:
- "Communicating is the alpha and omega, the beginning and the end in developing a relationship with my child, so therefore it is exceedingly necessary that we do so."
- "If we can't communicate, what can we do? All is lost without conversational give and take."
- "The experts say abundant communication, with your child is essential to being a good parent, so therefore I have to find a way to establish a conversational base with my child."
- "How dreadful that two people living under the same roof cannot establish communication."
- "If we don't learn to communicate, we will never get to know each other and how catastrophic that would be."
- "What a horrendous crime I am committing by not exercising my parental responsibility of cementing communication with my child."
- "It is my responsibility to take care of any and all communication lags with my child, so therefore I must do so."

Permissive countering ideas about parent-child communications that allow a lightening up so that either (a) pressure will be taken off communication avenues or that (b) allow participants to more gracefully accept the fact that for now at least, improved communication is not attainable, include:

- "Making myself accessible to open discussions with my child does not control it."
- "I will respect my child's right to have the privacy of her own thoughts."
- "Perhaps if I nag less about the avenues of communication they will become more traveled."
- "It takes two to communicate. The most I can do is follow; but if we are going to discuss, somewhere along the way it will be necessary for my child to take the lead."
- "Is communication really the answer to everything—or anything?"
- "Perhaps by making myself more tolerant of my child's decision not to talk to me, I will make it more attractive for her to begin to do so."

4. *Need for understanding.* This sought-after commodity is a rare bird, both in and outside parent-child relationships. Keep in mind that no one will likely ever understand you better than yourself. Perhaps the best way to invite someone to walk a mile in your moccasins is to not push for it. By insisting or commanding that you be understood, you push others further away. As with many illustrations in this chapter, the more you push your child in the direction you believe he "needs" to go, the more he is likely to pull in the other direction. Dictating a more complete relationship further alienates that possibility; often the more you persist, the more your child resists; the more you demand, the more your child gets himself out of hand. Rigid parental notions that bring on the emotional dependent need for understanding include:

- "If my own flesh and blood doesn't understand me, who can?"
- "I must gain and maintain my child's understanding; otherwise he will think less of me."
- "What bad things must I have done to bring about my child's boycotting an understanding of me?"
- "Children must understand their parents."
- "How else can a child learn except through an understanding of his parents' views and values?"

- "When my child doesn't understand me this increases the chances that he will betray my values—the ones he was brought up with!"

Challenging ideas that debate the parents' dire need to be understood include:

- "As with many dimensions of my relationship with my children, caring less without becoming uncaring are powerful words that give me more leverage and bargaining power as a parent."
- "When I wrongfully convince myself that I need my child's understanding, or anything else for that matter, I give him an emotional blank check and its use can result in my emotional bankruptcy."
- "My child's better understanding of me would be a highlight of my life—but not my life."
- "Understanding, especially from my child, would be a nice thing—perhaps even a great thing—but not a necessary commodity."
- "I won't die from my child's lack of undying understanding."
- "Demanding to be understood leads to desperately trying to control another human being. This lends itself to gaining less access to this pleasant resource.
- "The more I demand understanding, the more it is denied me."

5. *The need for never-ending agreement.* "Agree with me or you are unlovingly against me" is often the assumption of family members in conflict. Agreeing to disagree by accepting the nature of individual differences is an approach that challenges the agreement-upon-demand proposition. Agreeing to disagree without overdoing it helps members to comfortably be themselves rather than uncomfortably defending themselves.

The rush for never-ending agreement on command can be seen in these common rigid rules of family living:

- "If he really cared about those in his family he would see eye-to-eye with me."
- "If your own family doesn't agree, then who can?"
- "Love and agreement should be one and the same."

- "When my family members disagree with me, that proves that they are against me."
- "I always agree with them so therefore they must always agree with me."
- "I have to have my family's agreement because I can't stand being without such necessary social support."

Thoughts that pave the way for respect and encouragement of others' opinion are:

- "Agreement is great but hardly sacred."
- "All people are different, so it would be highly unlikely if we agreed on everything."
- "Everybody in this family is entitled to their and *not* my opinion."
- "It would be a boring world if we all agreed on everything."
- "Be glad we don't agree on everything, for if we did we would learn virtually nothing from one another."
- "Family living be a democracy rather than a dictatorship."
- "Welcome yourself (and others) to the real world of individual differences."

6. *The dire need for love.* When firmly, but nondemandingly embedded, love can be the hub of satisfying family relationships. However, there is no one-and-only place where love can be found. When family members' love for each other is viewed as a necessity, pressure is put on all concerned. If love is made into an essential element it will kill off goodwill and camaraderie. Narrow-minded family members' self-statements poison love's advantages. These statements block acceptance of the reality that just because people live under the same roof they don't necessarily love, honor, and obey each other.

   - "Love is a basic 'NEED' and if I can't even get it in my family, I'm doomed."
   - "My child's love for me = me."
   - "Without my family's love, I'm nothing."
   - "I can't get by in life without the love of each and every member of my family."
   - "What is wrong with me that my child doesn't show love toward me?"

- "Family love is a nonexpendable item, so without it, I'm expendable."
- "I hate my family for not generously providing me with my need for their love."
- "How could I ever make something of my life without my family's love?"
- "Gaining and maintaining my family's love is a desperate, urgent, all-important, bigger-than-life matter."

Statements that counter the insistence that love be freely given upon emotional demand include:

- "The more I push my family to repeatedly show love toward me, the more likely they are to pull in the other direction."
- "It would be better if I do not equate myself to my child's love for me."
- "I love my child very much, but I don't need him."
- "If I approach my child's love for me as a requirement, I'll give him a license to control me."
- "I can accept myself–preferably with but also without–my child's love."

7. *Insistence upon always and ever acceptance.* The ideal that "if others whom I've bonded with don't accept me, then I can't accept me" runs counter to emotionally healthy self-reliance. To set others' acceptance as a precondition for your own emotional well-being is to put yourself at the mercy of your child/ family member's decision to accept or to not accept you. Putting yourself on such a shoestring, like other emotionally dependent leanings, creates a breeding ground for hostility, i.e., "If you don't provide me with what I need from you, I'll resent you until the day that you die–and I hope it's soon."

Holding yourself emotionally hostage to your child's acceptance is seen in these faulty self-instructions:

- "What a miserable parent I must be to not be able to gain my child's acceptance."
- "If my child fails to accept me and my authority, he will be in trouble with authority figures all his life."

- "What will others think if word of my child's rebelliousness gets around?"
- "How shameful I am to be confronted with my own child's disregard."
- "What an absolute emotional horror it is when my child refuses to accept me–as I need him to."

Self-statements that can unshackle you from this too-strict alleged golden rule of parent-child relationships include:
- "When I don't gain undamning acceptance from my child, I don't have to damn myself."
- "Chances are my child's acceptance will ebb and flow and I am not the exception when it comes my way, nor am I unworthy when it doesn't seek me out."

8. *The need for a high-achieving child.* Many parents try to funnel their own life through their child's accomplishments and in doing so put a perfectionistic strain on family relationships. There is value to parents' understanding that they don't have to document themselves generally, and specifically through their child's achievements. Worshipping the God called child achievement is seen in frantic parental efforts to build their child's skills to a point of high tech performance, whether it be academically, athletically, musically, or artistically. Much emotional relief can ensue from refusing to scramble around sometimes from city to city, if not state to state, to display your child's genius. To want to assist in cultivating whatever strengths your child might possess is a thoughtful consideration; to think that you must see to it that these same skills be raised to a plateau that reflects "exceptionalism" can often create tension on all concerned. Efforts to promote your child's potential can be done for good and bad reasons; because you simply want your child to achieve to his full*er* potential vs. perfectionistically and desperately insisting that he do so to his full*est* capability. The latter may likely reflect deficiencies of self that you are attempting to mask, if not dissolve, through your child's abilities and achievements.

Self-statements that reflect an essential parental need for children to highly achieve include:

- "Getting my child to perform exceptionally well will reflect positively on me in the eyes of others, and I must not miss out on those exalted feelings that go along with such notoriety."
- "If my child performs and achieves better than his peers, this makes me a better parent and a better person."
- "I have to have a claim to fame in my lifetime and what better way to do so than through my child's accomplishments?"
- "I can justify my otherwise mediocre existence through the super achievements of my child."
- "I can't stand not being especially highlighted as the proud parent of an honor roll child."
- "What a great way to impress the relatives and God knows who else by producing a high-achieving child."

Countering beliefs that abolish parenting as an ego maneuver include:

- "I can encourage my child to achieve for his own best interest without thinking that his accomplishments put me a step above the rest of the human race."
- "My life can be a nice life of its own; I don't have to come in on my child's achievement shirttails."
- "I do not have to turn myself into a nut who has to impress others and be praised by them for any reason, including whatever accomplishments my child might gain."
- "I am, and will likely always be an imperfect parent of an imperfect child, not a perfect parent of a perfectly achieving child."
- "My own life has merits, with as few or as many achievements that go along with it."
- "I can stand on my own two feet, put one in front of the other as I move forward with my own life–with or without a high-achieving child."
- "If I make myself dependent on raising a high-achieving child, I will likely feel some resentment in the long run about such dependency."

9. *Need for feeling comfortable.* Parenting is not without its trials and tribulations; consequently, parents often don't feel in the peaches-and-cream comfort zone. Saying no to your child, when sometimes this "love word" often doesn't feel good; or making decisions about what to allow your child to do and not to do can be a queazy experience. Not knowing tomorrow's answers today regarding your child's plans and decisions is often associated with emotional turmoil. Not knowing the whereabouts or the activities of your child when he leaves with his peers can prove nerve-racking if you let it. Uncertainties about your child's physical and mental health can be an emotional balancing act due to your child's sometimes uncertain nature. Confusion, worry, fear, and anxiety are many times brought on in response to the above and other child and adolescent problems.

Emotionally dependent ideas that encourage upheaval about parental uncertainties include:
- "I have to know that everything will be fine with my child's future."
- "Parenting is supposed to feel enjoyable and be fun. I shouldn't feel so uncomfortable in being a parent, and I can't stand it when I do."
- "I should be able to make hard decisions about my child without feeling so uneasy about such matters."
- "Parenting has to be easy and comfortable and I have to make it so when it isn't."
- "I have to know the whereabouts of my child at all times because when I don't, bad things are more likely to happen."
- "I must have certainty, not uncertainty, security not insecurity, regardless of the unknown quantity that pertains to my child."

Hang on to your hat as a parent rather than let the wind of uncertainty blow it off. Maintaining some semblance of composure, or more fully accepting and/or tolerating the discomfort that goes with parenting, can be done by using these countering ideas:
- "Where is it written that parenting is supposed to be a bowl of cherries–without any pits?"

- "If I can't set aside or circumvent my own worries about my child, I can still forge ahead with my own life."
- "As long as I care about my child's future, I will be concerned about it, but I can avoid emotional consumption by not becoming dependent on controlling knowledge about my child's future and by not demanding that I be comfortable about whatever it might bring."
- "It is better if I understand and accept that the only way to feel calm and serene all the time is to not value anything, including my child's future."
- "It is better if I feel some level of trepidation and thus be more alert about decisions regarding my child, therefore I will be of keener mind in making them."
- "Many of life's endeavors that are worthwhile require effort and a high tolerance for discomfort. Why must parenting be different?"
- "Avoiding the trap of insisting that I be comfortable in parental efforts is likely to bring on the uncomfortable state that I wish to avoid."

Although appreciating the merits of becoming less dependent on decisions that only your child can make will likely not create happy parenting—every little bit can help. When emotional dependency is removed from the parenting equation, it loosens the bondage that holds parents hostage to the nine emotional-dependent dimensions described in this chapter. Pulling the plug on such dependency eliminates wishful, fraudulent thinking that prevents a balance of both power and emotions in parent-child encounters. This equal footing will likely equate to increased domestic quality of life, including the give and take that is absent from efforts grounded in fear and emotional dependency.

# Chapter 11

# With Kids Like That, You Don't Need Enemies

Parents need not look to their child, self, or society in search of special reasons to account for their offspring's problems and disturbances. As fate would have it, all humans rich or poor, red, yellow, black, or white, whether religious or nonreligious, regardless of functional or dysfunctional family upbringing, are born with remarkably fallible tendencies to overreact and to personalize life's happenings; to overgeneralize from one situation to the next; to be exceptionally demanding and perfectionistic, to name but a few inborn emotional cavities. Further, children as accidents waiting to happen bring their problematic potential to their family of origin and give expression to it within their family context. They use their parents to hang their emotionally disturbed hats on, which makes it very emotionally taxing for those in the parent role.

Children often insist:

1. That their parents take on all the favorable characteristics of their friends and other neighborhood parents, and seemingly won't settle for anything less than this perfectionistic ideal.
2. That no matter how hard the parent tries on the child's behalf that the child will still more likely than not strongly believe that his parents are trying to do him in.
3. That when the child feels upset, usually about being deprived of something, whether it be material goods, approval, or understanding, (a) it is the parents fault, and therefore, (b) the parent must change the situation and (c) then, and only then can the child feel happier. In short, parents practically always turn out to be a disappointment in the eyes of their children.

For those of you who have children and don't believe me—just
ask them and in no uncertain terms they will be very quick to
tell you that this is so!

To expect your child to routinely display such fingerpointing
antics in your direction can help to cushion the discontent of such
demands and blame. Children find it very convenient to blame their
parents and hold them accountable for matters of life that are out of
kilter. The trick for the parent is to not take such actions that insist
upon parental accountability for nearly everything that goes wrong,
and run with it. A large majority of parents come to their parental
decisions and responsibilities with good intentions, if not the right,
consistent, positive and negative consequential fashion. However,
to hear children tell it, their parents have nothing else better to do
than to intentionally make their life miserable.

Given this "damned if they do" and "damned if they don't"
double-bind dilemma, what is a parent to do? When almost every
goodwill effort on the part of the parent is followed by resistant
critical skepticism by the child, a combination of inner emotional and
outer behavioral protection is in order. Using parental tact and tactics
that incorporate tough-minded ideas that prevent overreaction, combined with behavioral expressions designed to create a temporary
distance between you and your doubting Thomas offspring, can
cushion his or her sassy aberrations. Such inner and outer declarations will be illustrated in the following two-part sequence.

*Part I*—Parental self-instructional coping statements that provide a
perspective that goes beyond the momentary insistences and criticisms of the unhappy acting child. Such self-stated ideas can assist
the parent to overreact less and take less personally their child's beefs
and antagonisms, while in the process accept themselves more in
spite of complaints and accusations from their child-adolescents.

These include:

- "I need not unduly upset myself just because my child has a
  bad case of normal paranoia which at his age has him blindly
  thinking that I have nothing else better to do with my time than
  to stalk, balk, and thwart him."

- "Why must I be the one parent in the universe who is able to raise unwhining, minimal-complaining children?"
- "I do not have to put myself on trial with my children."
- "I do not have to provide opposition for my children when they make themselves my opponent."
- "This difficult time in my life and that of my child will eventually pass for both of us, and after all is said and done, perhaps we won't be happy ever after, but possibly happi*er*."
- "Don't go for the disapproving bait and just maybe he won't cast in my direction as much."
- "Don't fight fire with fire."
- "Keep in mind you're not going to reason him out of something that he hasn't been reasoned into."
- "Don't fuel up the fire."
- "Don't throw emotional gasoline on his fiery complaints."
- "It is better if I understand and accept that my child, like all humans, has tendencies to be persistently insistent."
- "Emotional slack, yes! Emotional disturbance, no!"
- "The enemy isn't so much my child, as it is my overreaction to my child's words and deeds."
- "I need not seek—desperately or otherwise—my child's approval because my life does not certainly depend on gaining it."

*Part II*—Outer protective expressions that can provide an emotional and behavioral respite from the wiles of child-adolescent conflict. These verbal responses make convenient a neutralizing, marshmallowing, buffering effect that can take the wind out of your child's sails, while discouraging the onset of mutual needless argumentation. All examples have in common the ideas of acknowledging some truth in the child's negative comment/accusation while making it a point to blend in with the flow of the verbal attack, rather than meet it head on. See Figure 11.1 for "what to say back" illustrations.

Failing to see that due to your child's remarkably fallible, imperfect manner that he is by nature fated to not only have an abundance of problems but also to attempt to give you some, can leave a parent with mixed feelings of hurt, anger, guilt, and shame. Accept that it is a fact of nature that your child will display many problems, often venting them upon you. This can be the beginning of emotional

FIGURE 11.1

| Child's Statement | Parent's Response |
|---|---|
| • "I'm going to run away from home." | • "It sounds like sometimes you don't like living here." |
| • "I hate both of you." | • "It sounds like you're angry at your parents." |
| • "You're (absolutely) wrong and I'm (absolutely) right." | • "You really feel strongly about your opinion." |
| • "This is not right." | • "I admire the strength of your convictions." |
| • "You always say no." | • "I sense you believe us to be unfair to you much of the time." |
| • "You never let me do anything." | • "It is frustrating to hear no for an answer." |
| • "Every time I try to get you to understand me, you don't." | • "It's no fun being misunderstood." |
| • "I'm the only one of my friends who can't go." | • "It's often no fun to be the only one in a lot of situations." |
| • "I know that you hate my guts." | • "It's frustrating to feel others dislike you." |
| • "Your rules and ideas are all outdated and old-fashioned." | • "It's hard to accept that sometimes, some people aren't able to keep up with the times." |
| • "You don't ever trust me." | • "It's annoying not to feel trusted." |
| • "You treat me just like a little baby." | • "Most people do not like to be treated in a way that reflects their age." |
| • "Why do you treat me like you do?" | • "It sounds like you have a lot of questions about our motives." |
| • "Why do I have to go to school? I don't learn anything there anyway." | • "Sometimes it's not much fun at all to be legally required to do something that you find useless." |

relief that leads to being able to more effectively manage the problematic behavior. Learning to coexist with your child's flaws will not automatically lead to friendship, but eventually will likely greatly increase the chances of developing a friendship with your child that will make it necessary to look for enemies if you are to have any.

Chapter 12

# Eating Humble Pie:
# Guaranteeing Your Child Opportunity
# Without a Guarantee of Success

To create a sense of humility about what one can and cannot do for another person is especially helpful when sizing up the realities of parenthood. These days, pressure is put on parents to guarantee that their children succeed at school, in a vocation, and God knows where else. Ideas that counter this parent-child pressure cooker can provide a more knowledgeable perspective based on reality, paving the way for greater emotional relief for all concerned. Realities that have a humbling effect on parents include:

- Due to limited human capabilities, children will often not succeed at a level that matches the parents' output and success expectations.
- Many children have motivational deficiencies and betray their parents' best efforts to instill in them the will to prepare and succeed.
- The round peg in a square hole syndrome. The direction the well-intended parent attempts to send the child in may not be compatible with the child's natural tendencies.
- The bell-shaped curve syndrome. We live in a competitive world where few succeed exceptionally well in any field of endeavor. Most of us do not possess spectacular abilities. Instead we fall someplace in the mediocre range.
- The chance factor. As talented as your child might be, and as much as you may direct and nourish his skills, he will still

need to be in the right place, at the right time to succeed above par. Some of the greatest novelists, musicians, athletes, inventors, etc., did not live to see the fruits of their talent appreciated by the masses for this reason.

- The peer group factor. Regardless of how well you may have taught your child to think for himself, he may still cave in to peer pressure to engage in activities that he has been taught by you to avoid. Many good ideas and constructive efforts have been lost due to fear of peer ridicule. It would be wise for parents to accept and prepare for the reality that their child can be highly influenced by someone other than themselves.

- The cultural emphasis on the convenience factor. Children are affected by cultural messages that promote leisure excesses—that the way to lead a meaningful life is to lie on the beach 24 hours a day and do nothing. Taking the easy way out by worshipping the Gods called ease, convenience, and comfort causes child-adolescent motivation to fall by the wayside. After all, if I can get something for nothing and gain instant gratification, why should I learn how to work and wait for feelings of comfort? I can get similar feelings via more short-range, appealing methods, e.g., ride a dirt bike rather than walk, ride a jet ski rather than swim, watch endless television rather than think, flick on the stereo rather than pursue a hobby, click away at video games rather than organize a playground activity with friends.

- The human condition. Without any help from their parents, peers, or culture humans establish an affinity for comfort and then will invent ideas that support that yearning. For instance, perhaps the biggest myth of all time is that "it is easy to take the easy way out." Your child, just like anyone else's may adopt this faulty notion in spite of your efforts to try to instill in him a philosophy of effort.

Parents would do well to consider these eight pieces of humble pie, otherwise their unrealistic expectations may come crashing down on them. To sidestep this emotional fallout, parents can identify, review, challenge, and act against the irrational ideas that cause them to insist on a fair return on efforts on their child's behalf. Such off-base thinking is illustrated in the faulty notion: "If I provide my child with many of life's advantages and do many of the right things on his behalf, then naturally his future success must follow." Right? Wrong! Because you create abundant opportunity for your child in no way ensures abundant success. The world doesn't run in orderly cycles and consequently what goes around *doesn't* come around. There is often no payback, at least none that can be taken for granted. The previous faulty belief is challenged by the following series of ideas:

- "Though I gain pleasure and comfort in attempting to provide opportunity in my child's life, there is no assurance that I will find pleasure and comfort in the aftermath of my efforts."
- "Giving my child opportunity and seeing a successful return on such provisions are two different things. It is better to see and accept from the start that the two don't necessarily meet into one."
- "Having a sense of humility for what I can and cannot do for my child is wisdom to be relished."
- "Where is it written in granite that guaranteeing an opportunity for an individual also guarantees his or her success?"
- "There is no universal mandate that I will naturally see my child's success being guaranteed as a result of my presentation of opportunities."
- "Eating humble pie can taste good, especially when it eliminates pressure by allowing me to accept what I can't change."

Most important of all, the original irrational idea can be acted against. The best way to change an irrational idea is to act against it. This particular false idea can be overturned by application of the following tactics:

1. *Stay out of the way.* Provide your child with the various resources and remedies you have, then back off and let nature take its course. Beyond that you will likely end up trying to do your child's work for her in a futile attempt to guarantee her success.
2. *Don't force the issue.* Enough is enough! Pushing your child in the direction of the success you kindly had in mind may not

allow him to follow his natural bents, resulting in a you-push, he-pulls tug of war.

3. *Get a life.* Once you have done as much as you can to provide your child with the raw materials for his success, don't try to complete his project for him. Instead, look to yourself and your own unfinished projects, goals, and desires. Pursue them, thus you will stay out of your child's way and not try to do for him what only he can do for himself. You will also register and enjoy your own ambitions.

4. *Look for worthwhile causes to reinvest your leftover support and contributions.* Assuming you have not become exhausted from trying to present your child with golden opportunities in route to success, scan the community and see if there are not other ways you can satisfy your thirst for helping people. For example, do volunteer work for the Salvation Army, become a Big Brother/Sister, take on the responsibilities and opportunities of becoming a foster parent, volunteer at a nursing home, or devote yourself to animal rights principles.

5. *Survey the realities of the territory.* Look at the hard luck stories. Scan the front page of the newspaper, observing stories of those who have been able to guarantee their child opportunity but whose child's life has vastly betrayed the parents' hoped-for success.

6. *Humor yourself.* Laughing at yourself not only provides a protective refuge from your disappointments but also is a signal to yourself that you will prevail and endure this sometimes difficult time of your life without turning it into a disaster. Laugh about your child's goof-ups, to increase lightening up rather than tightening up, and tolerance rather than disgust. Self-statements such as "Damn me and my child for not making more out of opportunity," will lead only to emotional upset.

7. *Be transparent.* Talk to supportive others, including your mate if you have one. Discuss your ability to lead your child to water, create a little thirst in her, and your deficiencies in getting her to take a drink of the water. Such openness can provide emotional relief, especially when shared with someone who has had similar frustrations.

8. *Accept the paradox as part of the grand scheme of life.* There are many things that don't add up in the final analysis but were expected to be more congruent at the beginning. Being philosophical about these incongruities can help to pave the way toward moving in the direction of bigger and better things in your life.

Participating in your parenting role is a lot like participating in a democratic society; the better part of such a society assures its participants opportunity but because of life's impartial, objective nature it cannot guarantee success. Also, humans are not born equal, though they are born free (willed). They can work with opportunities presented to them and sometimes they will be able to accomplish what is in their long-range best interests; sometimes they will not be up to reaching such heights. A ten-year-old whom I recently saw for psychotherapy had engaged in sexual perpetration against a much younger child. After some discussion with him and his mother, which centered around putting more emphasis on correcting the problem in the future rather than condemning himself in the present, the mother asked, "How can I get him to not be so hard on himself?" I replied, "I don't think you can get him to do too much of anything, but what you can do is to invite him to more fully accept himself in spite of his bad, noncondoning actions." My response was part of a more general principle that I have attempted to highlight in this chapter: Wise parents will realize that there is only so much they can do to promote their child's success. Opportunities do not come with a guarantee of success. It is better for the child to be allowed to fail or succeed on his own.

Chapter 13

# Why Treat Children the Same
# When They Are All Different?
# Individualism Reconsidered

To enter parenting with an allowance for individual differences in offspring creates a more flexible, well-thought-out venture which in turn leads to emotional and behavioral harmony between parents and children. One size doesn't fit all in matters of family conduct toward one another. Just as forcing the wrong size shoe on one's foot can be painfully pinching, so too can forcing the same rules, expectations, allowances, and limitations on different children result in a lot of squeaking—if not squawking—from both the fitter and wearer. On the other hand, if the shoe fits, buy the other one and test out a philosophy of individual differences to see if you get favorable results for your relationship efforts. This chapter will suggest that one of the best ways to influence children is not to tell them that they are expected to follow one another, but to accept the option of following themselves.

A common error of parents is to try to make all their children out of the same mold, as if they were clones of one another. Such efforts go against the grain of human variance and distinctiveness. Examples of individual differences in children include:

- Some children require closer supervision by their parents, otherwise they stray off the beaten path in their relationships with the law, school, food, alcohol, money, etc. Creating a high level of structure is essential in avoiding trouble for *some* children.
- One person's cup of wine is another person's poison. The same structure and close supervision that is helpful for one

child will discourage the creativity of a more free-spirited child.

- Some children benefit from praise and other forms of positive reinforcement because they are by nature more easily conditioned. Without such pats on the back certain children find it difficult to motivate themselves toward constructive ends.
- Some children are less outwardly conditionable and the praise that pleases one child may cause a "spoiling affect" in another. Such a child often finds reinforcement within him or herself and left to his or her own recognition will simply feel good for a job well done without outside recognition.
- "Give him an inch and he will take a mile" may reflect one child's limit setting. With such a child it would be better if rules were applied in a strict, exacting, more inflexible manner, because if you don't he will likely see the loophole and run toward it headfirst. Stick to your disciplinary guns. There is little, if any room for compromise with this limit-testing child.
- Another child might not be so quick to take all she can get thus allowing room for compromise without fear that the child is going to take the family store. Proposals that reflect bending without breaking can be freely negotiated and undertaken without concern that this child will take advantage of your goodwill.
- Some children will find their own way socially without the formal benefit of peer group activities–scouts, band, Little League, choir, etc. These children have social instincts that don't require planned activities. In fact, if you try to impose such social structures into their routine they will not enjoy, and may openly balk at such "forced socialization."
- A different child may not be as free spirited in seeking out peer companionship and can use an added opportunity if not an extra push toward peer development. Sending him to camps for instance, can help him develop socially and become a less inhibited child.
- One child may require parental help with homework if she is to pull through grammer school. Due to natural "academic disinclinations," (meaning she seems allergic to school), nightly review of the homework with good communication monitoring between parents and teachers is suggested.

- Another child in the same family may find formal education requirements to his liking and consequently will instantly and instinctively take the lead in accelerating and excelling academically.
- One child will react to peer pressure by melting like butter in the sun in the face of it. A child who is naturally "soft" on what his peers think to the neglect of his own issues and answers could benefit from the parent looking over his shoulder periodically to peek at what might be going on. Parental awareness of the child's suspicious activities that could be leading to drug and/or alcohol experimentation does not guarantee that such activities will be stifled. However, unless the child is made aware that the parent is suspicious, it is less likely that such self-defeating conduct will be squelched before it becomes habit.
- Another child may be more inclined to naturally follow his own nose in not allowing himself to be motivated by powerful peer persuasion. Openly suspecting such a child of wrongdoing may damage the parent-child trust relationship. In fact, such an independent child might feel disappointed, if not insulted, by such a suspicion.

What most of these contrasting pictures of parenting guidelines reflect is a distinction between a high-maintenance child and a low-maintenance child. One child may require more parental guidance than a self-sufficient sibling, who may naturally behave in a way that leads to long-range happiness and success. Some children seem to instinctively take a long-range view of life. They are content with making short-run sacrifices for long-run gains, accepting present pain for future success. Others, also instinctively, choose to feel good now, at the risk of disadvantaging themselves the rest of their lives. They hold themselves hostage by their natural inclinations to act against their best interests.

The challenge of parenthood is to try to determine which sort of high- or low-maintenance child life has given you and whom you are forced to deal with. The suggested goal is to honor and to have a decent respect for individual differences between children, especially when they come from the same brood. Such an honest, realistic distinction allows flexibility in relating to offspring. Some can benefit from special favors and allowances whereas some will take advantage of them. Whatever measure, standard, or expectation that seems to fit this child is what would be best to apply, rather than the more confining view that one size fits all.

To anticipate complaints from the application of these individualized parenting methods is to be prepared for such nagging dissention. Examples of barbs that will likely be thrown your way by the odd-child-out, who isn't able to control for the advantages given to his or her siblings, include:

- "Johnny can do it; why can't I?"
- "It's not fair that she can go but I can't."
- "You trust him but you don't trust me."
- "If she can do it, I should be able to too."
- "If you loved me as much as you love him, you would buy me one too."
- "She gets everything that I don't get."
- "If I have to come in early, he should too."
- "She can hang around with anybody she wants, but you pick my friends."
- "How come my curfew is earlier than his?"
- "The same rule should apply to all of us."
- "You always compromise with her, but never with me."
- "You always make me do my homework, but you never tell him to do his."
- "You're always talking to my teacher about my homework but you never do about hers."
- "You treat me like a baby, and him like a grownup."

These verbal curve balls are designed to put the parent on trial so as to explain and explain some more. The parent can remind him/herself of the following coping ideas that prevent such courtroom procedures. Otherwise the parent may become emotionally dependent on the child's understanding.

- "My children are individuals why treat them differently?"
- "Although I may subject myself to my child's criticism by treating him differently, I would rather do what I think is best than what he thinks is best."

- "This is not a courtroom and I am not on trial."
- "I hope my child doesn't think that just because I treat him differently, doesn't mean that I don't love him. However, I can't control what he thinks."
- "Different strokes, praise, rules, and regulations for different folks."
- "No two things and no two people are alike, so what is the sense of treating them as if they were?"
- "One child's cup of tea is another child's poison—and I can poison my parenting by not appreciating that fact."
- "My children are obviously not two peas in a temperamental and behavioral pod. The sooner I recognize that, the better off we will all likely be."
- "A decent respect for individual differences between children sometimes causes parent-child relationship strain—but for a good reason."
- "To have a decent respect for individual differences between my children is one of the most decent things that I as a parent can do."

Without reconsidering individual differences you will likely encounter considerable problems in parenting. Treating children all the same does not allow you to accept the realities of individual differences. Not treating children all the same is not only a new way of approach to your relationships with your children, but may well be a more respectful, considerate way of approaching someone who is not only different from you but different from others who just happen to be living under the same roof.

Chapter 14

# Aspire and Inspire: Do It Yourself, Hire Someone Else To Do It, Forbid Your Child To Do It

It is the forbidden fruit that often motivates children. They will often want to do or learn the opposite of what their parents want them to do or learn. The more strenuously parents make requests of their child, e.g., do your homework, clean your room, limit your telephone calls, do the dishes, get to bed, often the less likely the child will take responsibility for keeping with the directive. Parental belaboring of these requests often has a paradoxical effect because practically all children search for control factors so that they can increase their chances to get what they want–precisely when they want it. To have the means to control their parents is often at the top of childrens' lists of priorities. When parents make their child's obedience into a sacred matter, *less* obedience is likely to be forthcoming. When the parent communicates to the child, "My satisfactions in life are largely dependent upon your willingness to honor and obey my requests–and I'm miserable when you don't," the child will likely take this bargaining chip and use it against the parent by refusing to cooperate. Such obstinacy can be better dealt with by abruptly turning away from such refusals, combined with some consequential hell for the child to pay for his oppositionalism.

It is almost as if the parent would gain more cooperation by instructing the child *not* to do what the parent desires him to do! Some parents actually try this paradoxical approach with periodic success. For example, a parent who wants his contrary-acting child to eat the peas that he is stubbornly refusing to, may *occasionally* find that the child actually eats the peas. However, such trickery and manipulation is seldom effective, works mainly with lesser intelligent beings, is somewhat dishonest, but worst of all has the net effect of reinforcing the child's oppositionalism. The parent wins the battle but looses the war because the child's oppositionalism is strengthened. The child believes that his obstinacy won out because he did the opposite of the parent's request—and he will likely continue to use such opposing tactics in the future. What appears to be the solution is really a strengthening of the problem—the same oppositional hearse with an even bigger license plate.

Rather than pleading with your child to fulfill simple responsibilities, change your thinking and consequently modify your response to such contrary behavior.

1. *Attitude change.* Remind yourself of some of the following coping statements designed to provide emotional slack and increased clearheadedness in managing your child's annoying behaviors:

- "Care less without becoming uncaring."
- "If it's going to be, it *doesn't* have to be up to me."
- "Save your breath and breathe easy."
- "I can lead a horse to water but it is *not* my responsibility to make him drink."
- "Be moderately concerned, not extremely consumed."
- "Stay involved—but don't entangle yourself."
- "It is better not to forget the value of having a sense of humility for what I can and can't do for my child."
- "I cannot transplant attitudes of ambition into my child's head nor feelings of motivation inside his gut."
- "Try to do what you can, but not overdo—otherwise your child may have you over a barrel."
- "I can invite and encourage my child to make the right, cooperative decisions—but that is as far as my helpfulness can extend."
- "By trying to do my child's motivational work for him I increase the chances of eventually creating resentment toward my child."

- "Share your life and your expectations with your child, but don't sacrifice your life for her."
- "Stop trying to sell your child a used car he doesn't want."
- "Don't try to reason your child out of something she hasn't been reasoned in to."
- "If I wear my fingers to the bone pleading my case for cooperation, I'll end up with bony fingers."
- "Sad that my child doesn't often cooperate—but not tragic."
- "Disappointments in my child's cooperation do not constitute disasters."

2. *Behaviorally it would be better to:*
   a. Simply state your request to your child, i.e., "I would like you to take out the garbage by 6:00 p.m."
   b. If there have been past squabbles regarding the garbage not being taken out on time, explain what negative happening will occur if the garbage isn't taken out on time and what positive happening will occur if it is taken out on time. For instance, "For each five minutes that the garbage isn't taken out on time you will be docked twenty minutes of curfew time for the next week, and if the garbage is taken out by 6:00 p.m. your curfew and allowance will remain intact."
   c. Apply enormous detachment. This is as far as you can take the motivational ball for your child. Provide him with a negative consequence that will likely displease him enormously and a positive consequence that will likely please him enormously. Then back off, enormously detach yourself and let him decide by which set of consequences he wishes to live by. Your job is not to try to do mission impossible by making the decision for him, but rather to enforce the previously stated consequential expectations. By creating the conditions that force your child to decide one way or the other you are preparing him for future life choices that require him to decide which options contribute to his long range happiness and survival and which don't. Providing a child with decision-making opportunities is a gift of much benefit.

This direct, consequential, practical application of cognitive and behavioral principles is a straightforward approach that encourages learning of and collaboration with your child concerning obedience expectations. Paradoxical intention–forbidding your child to do something in hopes that he or she will do it–is an indirect, meager, last-resort effort to motivate your child when all else fails. The precise teaching factor is abandoned in favor of such a deceptive approach. Rather than forbidding your child to forsake the forbidden fruit and scolding him unendingly when he doesn't, your chances of success may be much greater if instead you aspire to inspire him by explaining the principles of negative and positive reinforcement that will be applied according to whether he toes the mark or not.

Chapter 15

# The Real ME-Coy:
# Implications of Fraudulently
# Living Your Life Through Your Child

Being yourself with your social group rather than proving your-self to your social group is a lofty mental health ideal. To deter-mine not to define, rate, judge yourself by anything about or a part of your existence is a rarity. Perhaps you can count on one hand the number of people you have met in your lifetime to whom "what you see is what you get" applies. Self-proving is allowed to get in the way of more authentic self-presentation. The search for a sub-stitute for self and for one's capabilities often finds its way to the parenting role. Overcompensation—using one's child to compen-sate, make up for, or substitute for everything the parent hasn't achieved or gained in life is a common problem that has negative implications for all concerned. Defining and addressing these problems is the subject of this chapter.

Most parent problems are ego problems, problems of self-evalu-ation, i.e., "I am my parenting" rather than "I am a parent. I do my parenting but I am not my parenting." Too frequently parents expect their parental role to justify themselves, especially if they haven't measured up to their ideal expectations of life. Being dis-appointed not only in their life, but in themselves as human beings, they often look to their children to document their identify. This puts a lot of pressure on all concerned. The child feels pressure because he/she is expected to be everything the parent wasn't—scholar, athletic, beauty queen. The parents experience tension in the process of attempting to force the child to mirror what they believe they lack in themselves. With such pressure being applied it is difficult at best to function in a free-wheeling, emotionally healthy manner. To attempt to mold offspring in one's own idealized self-image is to attempt to stifle the child's natural inclinations and to create much family conflict and bickering. The result is a pushing and pulling match–the more the parent pushes the child in the "be like everything I wanted to be" direction, the more stress and strain will take its toll as the child pulls in the opposite direction. The child and the parents both lose in this self-proving scuffle. The child, due to the parents' prodding, finds it difficult to find his individualized niche. The parent gives up the search for his own goals in life–instead shadowing his own ambitions with his child.

It is important for parents to understand that if their child turns out to be a great person and/or a scholar that this does not make them wonderful parents, or if the child falters they are not terrible parents. It is important for parents to learn how to avoid the self-measurement trap, i.e., "I am my parenting." By fully accepting themselves as they are rather than trying to live their lives via the expectations they have of their children, they unshackle themselves from the burdens of make-believe, fraudulent family living. A solid beginning to moving away from this invisible dependence on children is to identify and then counter the irrational beliefs that set this overcompensation pattern in motion. Table 15.1 is a list of those irrational beliefs (IBs) that lock parents into this child-dependent pattern and those countering beliefs (CBs) that allow them to move away from such dependency.

Using your child's life to justify your own is a poor substitute for seeking your own independent experiences while further exploring your own boundaries. It is emotionally healthy to want what would be better for children, but not just because their actions emulate your own unrealized values and ambitions. Desiring that your child experience success is to be encouraged, but do not use such victories to compensate for your own alleged shortcomings.

## TABLE 15.1

<u>IB</u>

1. "I must have something to show for my life; if not my children, then what?"

2. "I've never amounted to much, but maybe I can still squeeze in some self-worth through my childrens' achievements."

3. "I am going to get my children to be everything I wasn't."

4. "You only go around once and if I can't at least see my children accomplishing what I didn't, my life would be a total loss twice over."

5. "My children must excel—or else others will think less of me, especially since they can see all that I've failed at."

6. "How else can I prove myself if not through the successes of my children?"

7. "To have a high-achieving child provides me with something to flaunt in front of the others."

8. "When I die nobody will know me, save through the accomplishments of my children."

<u>CB</u>

1. "Why must I have to document my existence and my attempts to enjoy it?"

2. "I am not less worthy for not living up to my expectations of myself, and neither will I be holier than thou if my children live up to what I didn't."

3. "Pushing my children to achieve and perform as I didn't will only encourage them to oppose me. It is better to take a view that encourages each of us to be ourselves."

4. "It would be nice if my kids could exceed my performance standards, but my life does not depend on such outcomes."

5. "To ask my children to be like I wasn't isn't fair to them and prevents my own life from being more free-standing."

6. "To begin with, there is no evidence that I must prove myself either through my children or my children's good works."

7. "What would be the point in playing psychological games via my children or anything else for that matter?"

8. "When I die I will no longer even know myself, so what is the point of my insistence upon notoriety?"

TABLE 15.1 (continued)

| <u>IB</u> | <u>CB</u> |
|---|---|
| 9. "To have been on this earth with nothing to show regarding my childrens' achievement patterns would openly document to myself and to others my secret sense of self-depreciation." | 9. "I will make myself better off by taking on a philosophy of 'self-judgments have I none'." |
| 10. "I absolutely have to find and impress upon my child my lost potential—that way both of us can define ourselves as being successful." | 10. "I know of no way possible that I can transplant my lost ambitions into my child's head and to try and stuff such goals into his head and down his throat will only serve to distance us from one another." |

Efforts to make do through your child's life rather than your own seldom materialize because:

1. *You can't turn back the clock and do now what was or wasn't done then.* To try to make up for such lost time leaves you searching for something that doesn't exist—reclaiming the past with a different ending.
2. *Children's oppositional tendencies.* Due to strivings for independence children will often pull away from parental pressures. The child may unknowingly be cutting off his nose to spite his face but while spiting himself will often push himself in the opposite direction of the parents' strong suggestions.
3. *Nonexistence of ambition and motivational transplants.* Mission impossible is to try to head someone in an opposite direction. A team of wild horses and a set of parents combined cannot accomplish this task. To expect children to want to be what you weren't is to disregard their individual inclinations. Such forceful efforts to get the child to camouflage her natural bents and to instead take on your aborted ambitions will likely fail.
4. *Whatever the decoy the child is expected to play, it is a pale*

*substitute for the real McCoy.* Even though the parent has fallen short of original ambitions, at least such shortcomings constitute accurate, valid reality rather than an artificial cover-up. There is value in being true to yourself and accepting your failings as well as yourself. This is perhaps the saddest part of parents' expecting their child to substitute for their own deficiencies. Such efforts imply a lack of an important dimension to the human condition–unconditional self-acceptance. If parents truly accepted themselves along with their goal-achievement shortcomings, they would be much more inclined to leave well enough alone in child rearing. Instead of trying to apply this "your life for mine" trade-off, parents can use their past failings to work on their own mental health by accepting themselves with their flaws, while making it more convenient and less conflicting for the child to be himself. It is hazardous to not separate the "me" from the "you" in parent-child relationships by using your child as a decoy instead of accepting the real ME-Coy that exists in both of you.

Chapter 16

# Doing *to* Your Child
# vs. Failing to Accept
# What Can't Be Done
# *for* Your Child

I have met exceptionally few parents whose goal in life was to
banish their child's emotional well-being, trying diligently to purposefully do them in; I have met many parents who after talking to
them I couldn't understand why they didn't want to do their
child(ren) in! A majority of parents have good intentions but
because of their difficulty in accepting what they cannot do for their
child are unable to back up their positive intentions with the right
disciplinary, ignoring and/or supportive, affirming methods. Even
when in the throes of yelling, nagging, or otherwise trying to corral
their child, they maintain a sense of love for and confidence in their
targeted child. At other times what is hidden behind such negative
parental antics are caring parents whose harsh words are their way
of giving vent to their fears; they are afraid that unless they robustly
intervene their child will cause himself severe harm. The last objective behind the parents' emotional smokescreen is to prevent harm
to their child. If they didn't care for their child, think she could do
better by gaining advantages for herself, and weren't afraid that her
oppositionalism and/or underachievement might eventually do seri-
ous harm to her long-range goals and ambitions, they wouldn't
bother to lift a finger on her behalf. Such roundabout encouragement may not appear very constructive, but is really a futile attempt
to persuade the child to concentrate on her potentials and capabilities.

This chapter is designed to encourage and cultivate a better understanding of what often lies beyond parent-child conflicts. Such proposals can then be used as vehicles to better lubricate and take pressure off family members' interactions. When parents begin to better understand their own favorable intentions and when children begin to appreciate the honest, well-intended efforts of their parents, the stage is set for fostering a more permissive domestic relationships. This realistic appraisal points to the fact that parents support their child's best interests and enables parents and children to consider the advisability of hanging together rather than hanging separately.

Approach parent-child conflicts in the spirit of emotional containment rather than overreaction, goodwill rather than unforgivingness, compromise rather than oppositionalism. This requires a review of the problems so that one does not attempt to solve problems without knowing what they are. When parents fail to accept what they can't do for their child in terms of happiness, more rational thoughts, and behavior, complications arise that create problems for all concerned. The following will sum up what the problems are for the parent as well as for the child, the irrational beliefs (IB) that trigger such upsets and difficulties, and countering self-instructions (CST) that serve as remedial mechanisms.

*Parental problem #1.* Self-rating, self-judgments, self-evaluations.
**IB**–"I must/have to find solutions to my child's bad problems or I am bad. After all, I not only do my parenting–but I am my parenting."
**CST**–"I want to do what I can do to steer my child away from bad, self-defeating behavior, but I am not bad when I am unable to do so. After all, I do my parenting but I am not my parenting."

*Parental problem #2.* Low frustration tolerance (LFT).
**IB**–"I absolutely can't stand to see my child make mistakes so I must disguise my discomfort by doing his life discovery work for him."
**CST**–"Watching my child make errors is not a pleasant sight, but it is bearable, and the longer I bear my discomfort the less likely that I will jump into his life in a manner that will merely make matters worse."

*Child problem #1.* Grandiosity, center-of-attentionism, self-centeredness, demandingness.

IB—"My parents and the world owe me the things that I miss, including eternal bliss and it's terrible when they don't provide my worldly requirements."

CST—"There are many things in life that I want, and if I want them enough, better that I strive for them, rather than helplessly whine and complain about their absence."

*Child problem #2.* Low frustration tolerance, impatience, avoidance of responsible behavior.

IB—"My parents should provide gratification for me because I'm a minor who deserves the good things in life. I can't stand to wait for them, or for someone else to provide them—or heaven forbid—have to work for them myself."

CST—"Granted, waiting is no fun but I can tolerate both playing the waiting game or getting my rear in gear as will likely be required if I am to gain the advantages I desire."

Who causes more problems, is it the crook or the well-intended honest person who bungles the job due to poor methods? By the same token, which family is going to suffer from more emotional strain: the rare ones in which the parents intentionally try to do something bad to the child, or those in which the parents fail to see and/or accept what they can't do for the child—or are both equal? Sharing your life with your child can be a terrific thing; sacrificing yourself as a parent isn't so good. Parenting is like most relationship endeavors—it is nice to give and receive. It may be a long time before your children appreciate or understand the rhyme and reason behind your limit-setting declarations. Try to appreciate the wisdom that distinguishes between doing *to* vs. failing to accept what you can't do *for* your child. See if it isn't one of the biggest favors that you can ever do to *and* for one another.

# Chapter 17

# Is Behavior Gone Unnoticed Really Less Likely to Occur? What the Behavior Modifiers Fail to Tell You

'Twas the night before my then ten-year-old son Billy's spelling test, and not a creature was stirring–not even Billy–in regard to studying for the test. Being privy to his special interest in shooting billiards, I proceeded to sit him down and give him an offer that I thought he couldn't refuse. I said, "I'll tell you what, Billy. We'll study for tomorrow's spelling test in Mr. Murphy's class, and if you get between 80 and 90 on it you can shoot billiards for one half hour at the pool hall. If you get between 90 and 100 on it you can shoot for a full hour." Billy replied, "You cheapskate." So much for the theory that says behavior is shaped by its consequence. Parents are told to praise their child when he behaves, and ignore him when he misbehaves. Simple enough, huh? But what happens when the county district attorney comes knocking at your door with the intention of accusing you of neglect?

Behavioral management/modification techniques can be instrumental in helping motivate some children some of the time. However, children respond differently to parental reinforcement efforts; some children will do anything for an M&M and others will tell you to shove it. Some kids will swear by your rewards–and some will swear at them! This is because some children are more suggestible, reinforceable, and conditionable than others. Although every decision has a consequence, children's behavior is not so much shaped by its consequences as by the thinking of the child who is experiencing the consequences. Until 1955, when Albert Ellis founded

Rational Emotive Behavior Therapy (REBT), most people believed the S/R (stimulus causes response) theory. However, REBT advocated a different direction in human thought and emotion by pointing out that between the S and the R is the "O," the organism or individual who mediates between the two. When offered an incentive or provided with a reward for constructive conduct, one child might agree that this motivator agrees with him and say to himself:

- "This is an opportunity I can't pass up."
- "I'll try as hard as I can to act good so I get the prize."
- "I'll feel so good after I earn it."
- "The bigger the reward, the harder I'll work."
- "I'll do it to get what I want."
- "I won't do it because I'll be punished if I do."
- "I'm afraid of what will happen if I disobey."

Another, less reinforceable child might look at the same reward or punishment quite differently, taking a less fascinated view, concluding that such reinforcers are only minimally interesting if not totally insignificant for the purposes of gaining his attention.

Such mavericks may instead say to themselves:

- "Who needs it?"
- "I'll outlast them and get it anyway."
- "I'm not going to let them get me to give in!"
- "I can take whatever punishment they can dish out (standing on my head)."
- "They can't make me do anything."
- "I'll show them."
- "They can't control me."
- "The harder they punish me, the more stubborn I will be."
- "I don't have to do anything that I don't want to do."

When parents realize that different children will respond differently to the same stimulus, they can take some solace in admitting to themselves that perhaps it's not the solution to their child's difficulties that is not in order, but rather that the motivational problems their child has are simply tough ones. Such a realistic appraisal can help pave the way for parents to not take personally or take responsibility for their child's dilly-dallying, lethargic disposition. Nothing is foolproof, including behavioral tactics designed to get one's child to overcome her motivational deficiencies. There is the story of pickpockets being hung publicly to discourage pickpocketing. The surprise of the day was that while the hangings were going on right before the audience's very eyes, there were people in the same audience, of all things, picking pockets! The negative reinforcement was simply not getting through. Such illustration can be applied to raising the level of your child's inspiration *and* perspiration, regardless of the strength of either the positive or negative reinforcement applied. No one can push a person up a ladder unless he or she wants to go up to begin with. Helen Keller said, "Science has not found a remedy for the worst of evils–the apathy of human beings"–not even the behavior modifiers.

But be of good heart and head. Your child's good behavior is not less likely to occur because it was unnoticed, nor is bad behavior less likely to occur if left unnoticed. Understand and accept that for better or for worse, your child's conduct is not necessarily shaped by the consequences of your actions. Thus, you can free yourself from assuming responsibility regardless of how far your child does or doesn't dip into his motivational barrel. When you succeed in learning what the behavior modifiers fail to tell you, you accept yourself rather than assume that you are in ego heaven when your child complies with your standards or be tenured in ego hell if your child fails to live up to your saintly expectations. A problem with success is that learning is less likely to take place. Instead of waiting for behavioral experts to tell you about children's individual differences you can discover this for yourself. One measure of success is how you handle it–and you can succeed by learning the many exceptions to the "stimulus causing the response" rule to become a more well-rounded person as parent–in spite of what you have or have not been told.

Chapter 18

# Nature vs. Nurture
# in Children

The vast majority of people that you will meet in your life are for themselves and the values that express their nature, rather than against you—this includes your children. Realizing this can help you to take others' treatment of you less personally. Hostility and hurt can be neutralized when it is understood that others' expression of temperament and disposition is only natural toward anyone and would be displayed in a similar situation.

For better or worse it is difficult to stifle human potential. Humans simply head themselves in the direction of their genetic biases. Human potential may be temporarily arrested but it will eventually break through. Since nothing between any two people is ideal, frustrations and annoyances will frequently crop up in any parent-child relationship. When parents find their child is dissatisfied with them, they often take responsibility for such disenchantment by assuming that it is their child's upbringing. Parents believe they must have done something wrong regarding the child's nurture or upbringing, thus causing the child's misgivings about family relationships and/or life in general.

What parents often fail to realize is that because life is such a hassle, often dominated by frustration and irritation, and because their child is human, he or she is likely to escalate that frequent displeasure into a high level of upset. This tendency to blow up dissatisfaction into disturbance is a given of the human condition. Just because parents are the central context of the child's nurturing does not make them accountable for their child's emotional outcome. Realizing this can slacken differences and lead to more free-wheeling, permissive parent-child relationships. You can take the boy out of the country but you can't take the country out of the boy; by a similar token you can sometimes remove your child's dissatisfactions, but you can't take away your child's tendency to make himself disturbed in life circumstances that are less than perfect. You may be able to pacify him for a time, but it is unlikely you will be able to please him enormously and in doing so convenience his happiness indefinitely.

Your child, like anyone else, can remove or run from what she finds displeasing, but she can't hide from her natural tendencies to overreact and to personalize what she defines as unpleasant. Much emphasis is put on the child's nurture as a factor in personality development, to the neglect of her "disturb-ability"–her ability to disturb herself regardless of the quality of her life circumstances. Naturally, children will ordinarily behave better when a way is found to pacify or please them. You can spend much of your parenting years trying to do just that. Lots of luck, and it's likely you will need much of that! Or, you can accept that your child will be imperfect despite your best efforts to instill happiness and wisdom while exposing her to as many pleasant experiences as possible. When it comes to emotional disturbance, nature rules supreme. If the child doesn't overreact in her family of origin she will do so within a different compartment of her life. This revelation can dispel emotional sting when it seems as if your child is turning against you, but you realize instead that she is simply being herself.

Child rearing examples that reflect nature's biases include:

- Adopted males whose fathers had a criminal record have a higher rate of criminality than boys whose fathers have not been imprisoned for violating the law–even though in either case the boys never met their fathers!
- Children of adopted parents tend to take on the same eating habits as their natural parents–whom they have never met! Natural children raised in the same family and exposed to similar value systems, often turn out to be quite different.
- Adopted children raised by adoptive parents are often quite different than the natural children of their adoptive parents, even though raised in a similar manner.

- After the birth of their first child many parents believe their nurturing to be the primary factor in their child's personality. After their second child when they see the major differences between the first child and second child, parents often begin to appreciate the "hard-wired" (i.e., fixed) nature factor.
- Over the last 30 years that I have done psychotherapy I have come across perhaps hundreds of single custodial parents who tell me that their child has many of the characteristics, traits, and temperament of the noncustodial, absentee parent—whom the child has never met!
- I have seen a handful of parents who placed their child up for adoption at birth and many years later have sought out their natural child. Or, as more frequently occurs, parents have been sought by their birth child of many years ago. Parents were surprised when they discovered that their child was very similar to them in regard to temperament.

If these children in some of the above illustrations had been raised by their natural parents, a vast majority of experts and lay people alike would have concluded that the child's personality makeup was learned—that he is modeling what he saw—because children learn what they see. However, you are required to see behavior in order to copy it. If nurture or learning were the answer to everything in terms of understanding child development—all children would learn the same response from the same stimulus—which as some of these examples illustrate, does not occur. Yet, parents and counselors of parents continue to cling to the myth and mystique of nurture, especially being cared for tenderly as being an absolute, indispensable link to successful child rearing. This fallacy represents convenient thinking because there are so many (overlooked) exceptions to the nurture rule. The sad part of all of this is that given the alleged dominance of nurture parents begin to run scared, adopting a negative view of parenting and self. The parents may well be doing many of the "right" things but may be getting "wrong" results because of their child's inborn tendencies toward fallibility. To chalk up to nurture what can more accurately be attributed to nature is to set in motion a false premise, i.e., that children are against you and are being harmed by your nurture; that unless challenged and dissolved, a chain of misunderstandings will be set in motion that will further complicate or sabotage the best parental intentions.

Humans, including children, make themselves especially prone to the idea that "If I deem something to be good then I have to have it." Desiring certain pleasures or avoiding certain displeasures but not being able to gain or avoid them will result in nurture limiting, frustrating, depriving, and inconveniencing the child, i.e., he can't have an extended curfew, cannot have a friend sleep over on a school night, cannot use the car, cannot escape an abusive life or family circumstance. The child's natural demanding nature that has him insisting and dictating what must and/or must not be will escalate the original frustration into a full-blown emotional disturbance. Nurture frustrates, nature induces disturbance by demanding that the beginning displeasure not exist. See Figure 18.1 for a descriptive flow of how children often exacerbate events, rupturing dissatisfaction into emotional disturbance.

Try as you may, it is unlikely that you will be able to create the ideal world for your child. Blaming your child's inevitable emotional and behavioral problems on yourself and your nurturing may be the fashionable, and seem the natural, most convenient, thing to do. However, encouraging yourself to do so will only appear to document that your child is against you rather than for him or herself. Worse yet, it will pit you against yourself, a natural, but not healthy thing to do. Rather than heed your own nature and blame yourself, compassionately and cushion your response to your child's misgivings. Give yourself some emotional slack as a parent—and don't look back!

FIGURE 18.1. Rational vs. Irrational Emotional Responses in Parent-Child Conflicts

| Child's belief that parental nurturing frustrates. | Accompanying rational, sensible ideas of the child that will contain the frustration(s): | Ideas brought into play that reflect the child's natural tendency to escalate preference into demand: | The parents' typically irrational, nonsensical ideas that piggyback off the child's demands: | Countering sensible beliefs of parents and/or child |
|---|---|---|---|---|
| • Child requests to: Use the car, own a gun, extend curfew, stay overnight at a friend's house, borrow money, etc.—some/all of which the parent says "no" to. | • "I wish my parents would be more cooperative and give in more."<br>• "It's always disappointing to hear no, but maybe next time they will be more favorable."<br>• "It's not the end of the world to be told no."<br>• "At least now I know." | • "I must have my own way."<br>• "I can't stand it when my parents refuse me."<br>• "I shall be miserable until my parents give in."<br>• "My parents have no right to refuse such simple requests of mine." | • "My child must not question authority or talk back in any way."<br>• "I can't tolerate and will not tolerate my child's complaints and arguments."<br>• "If I don't squelch my child's opposition immediately, it may get out of hand."<br>• "What a bad parent I must be for my child to talk to me in these disrespectful ways." | • "Others have a right to see things their way, not just my way."<br>• "I don't have to make such a big deal out of others' reactions."<br>• "Chill out."<br>• "Cool your jets."<br>• "Go easy."<br>• "Lighten up." |
| | Accompanying healthy emotional reactions<br><br>Disappointment<br>Frustration<br>Displeasure<br>Annoyance<br>Irritation | Accompanying unhealthy emotional reactions<br><br>Anger<br>Hurt<br>Betrayal | Accompanying unhealthy emotional reactions<br><br>Fear<br>Anger<br>Hurt<br>Betrayal | Accompanying healthier emotional reactions<br><br>Concern<br>Disappointment<br>Regret<br>Sadness<br>Displeasure |

Chapter 19

# Is Blood Really Thicker Than Water? Loyalty, Love, Obligation, and (Dis)Agreement in Family Relationships

Charles Dickens said, "Accidents will occur in the best-regulated families." Most families have a fair amount of mutual loyalty, love, and obligation; it just sometimes appears that they don't. This is because disagreement often enters the picture. All families do not automatically exhibit love, loyalty, obligation, and agreement. Family members betray one anothers' values about as much as any other group of people. The fact that family members often differ from one another in tastes, preferences, and value expressions is difficult for some to understand and even harder for many to accept.

To believe that bloodlines ought to transcend individual differences is to invite strained family relationships. This faulty belief promotes a personalized view of disagreements, i.e., "What is wrong with me that I can't get my family member to agree with me?" This guide will discuss (a) what family members really owe one another regarding agreement, (b) what their disagreements represent, (c) observations of common family bonds that often get lost in in-house fighting and feuding, (d) ideas for prevention of conflict and disharmony in family relationships.

"If you love me, you would agree with me," could be countered with, "If you loved me, you wouldn't disagree with me." Both of these statements are barking up the wrong tree since they imply that because people live under the same roof they are expected to be on the same wavelength. Believing that kinship is related to indebtedness will spark family disturbance through believing that family members owe each other unquestioned agreement, and to behave otherwise is an unpardonable sin. Goodwill between family members will increase if they can relinquish the idea that they must see eye to eye simply because they are family.

Disagreement among family members is the same as disagreement between people outside of families—the dissenter is building a case to support his or her values. Practically anyone, regardless of how disagreeable they act, are for themselves and their values rather than against you. When the shoe is on the other foot and you are doing the disagreeing, you are likely to be for yourself and not against the other. Opposing values differs from opposing people. Because someone balks at your ideas and labels them bad, this does not mean they are saying that you are bad. Try to corral the faulty inference that your family members have nothing better to do than to disagree with you.

Unfortunately, much of what is good in family connections goes unnoticed when members engage in dysfunctional thoughts about their observations and inferences. First, they observe their kin's disagreement; second, they become suspicious about the dissenter's motives, e.g., "He's against me"; "He hates me"; "She's trying to get me mad." Finally the disturbance chain is completed by concocting irrational beliefs about the original observations and inferences, e.g., "If he loves me, he shouldn't thwart me and my values"; "What kind of person would not be loyal to his own flesh and blood? A no-good betrayer, that's who"; "She must always agree with me. After all, we weren't brought up to be enemies"; "This is utterly horrid that my own family would have the gall to not agree with me." Getting past this dictatorial, intolerant thinking, and the hostile feelings it creates can reveal some deeply kept secrets out of which bonding relationships can be built. These include:

1. When questioned, especially alone, most family members will admit that there is no other place they would rather live than their current family residence.
2. Practically all agree that they would stick up for the others if they overheard them criticized by a third party.
3. If pursued, they usually will admit to and agree that in spite

of their contrary behaviors, they have a common goal of getting along better.

4. Although sometimes reluctant to admit it, they have hopes and expectations that they will survive and thrive together in the long run.

5. Even though as individuals they often believe they are getting the short end of the advantages stick, they often will admit that they could have done much worse, i.e., as a parent or child.

6. When prompted, they can usually identify what they like best about their family and the individuals in it.

7. Family members will acknowledge the activities they have enjoyed together.

8. They can highlight common enemies and hassles they have joined forces to combat.

9. They can identify what advantages there would be for family life if each stopped fighting fire with fire.

10. They are capable of posing a future controversial situation and discussing how it could be better handled.

11. Pledge a good thing to do when each doesn't get their own way.

12. Together, family members can identify thoughts that cause hurt and anger. These can be used as self-talk to prevent such dysfunctional feelings.

13. Family members can pinpoint emotions and behaviors each would like others to increase. Ask each other if this is reasonable and if each is willing to do so.

14. Discuss changes in their own conduct that would contribute to bigger and better things happening in the family.

15. Discuss things they are proud of about their family and the last time they bragged about it.

16. Admit that other family members don't have to change their behavior before each can better his or her own.

17. Highlight the happiest moment in their family.

18. Identify what it takes to encourage others in the family to laugh.

19. Point out improvements each has seen in one another's personal development.

20. Point out personality traits that make it easier for other family members to act kindly toward them.
21. Determine the best response when another family member doesn't say what one wants to hear.
22. Family members are capable of finding value to discussing: "What becomes of families like us? How do their lives turn out?"
23. Members understand and accept that other members don't have to admit they are wrong for life to continue peacefully.
24. They can affirm how they would like to be thought about and remembered by others in the family.
25. Members are aware and are willing to mention unique talents they notice in other family members.
26. They are willing to support the idea of family members' listening to each other more and how this can be better accomplished.
27. They are capable of identifying what they have learned from each other.
28. Family members are able to pinpoint a positive occurrence they noticed in their family within the week that they would like to see continued.
29. They can recall the nicest thing another family member did for them.
30. Members can complete the question, "we are lucky to be together as a family because. . . ."
31. They are able to discuss how each thinks their family is unique from any other.
32. Each member is willing to respond to, "What my family likes best about me being around is. . . ."

Loyalty, love, obligation, and agreement are often lumped together as "givens" of all constructive family relationships. This figment of imagination runs counter to the scientific evidence that people are not clones of one another. Accepting this and the following suggestions will go a long way toward accomplishing some of the acknowledgements previously stated in the service of more harmonious family living.

a. *Agree to disagree.* Nothing between humans is ideal, often far from it. Realize that you are going to differ at times but try to let these differences rest rather than debate them.

b. *Don't try to make others over.* Awaken yourself from the impossible dream of transplanting your values to another.

c. *Respect similarities and differences.* Entertain the possibility that your family has a common goal to increase the quality of your home life. Then, respect the fact that you each probably have different means of accomplishing this end.

d. *Seek responsible word precision.* Each would do well to begin analysis of their disturbance with, "I upset myself when I see what I don't like in others' conduct. Now how can I become less upset about such matters?" Rather than, "He/she gets me mad when he/she does not act in accordance with what I like." Take the position that reflects self-responsibility rather than the position that mirrors other blame.

e. *Don't go for the "misery likes company" bait.* Humans tend to want to share their unhappiness. When one member tries to tempt you to join him in his unhappiness be sure to decline the offer. Don't add fuel to the fire by taking on his contrary manner.

f. *Anti-exaggerate.* Statements such as "He always starts a fight"; "Everytime I try to be nice to him he doesn't act nice back"; "Never once has she been helpful," make it more difficult to accurately see what you are up against in terms of conflict and ill will.

g. *Respect others' fears.* Family members' attempts to control signal their fear of losing what they view to be requirements for survival, i.e., others' cooperation, understanding, approval. Anger is pressed into action to control and intimidate others to provide these alleged necessities that are thought to be lost. Rather than counterattack these feeble attempts to get beyond the misery equation, "others' opinions equals me," have compassion and respect for these efforts.

h. *Use constructive ways to get others' attention.* Be forthright in seeking others' acknowledgment but don't rant and rave, or be aggressive and abusive in doing so.

i. *Offer cooperative trade-offs.* As in life generally, constructive family living is often a series of exchanges in which people do things for one another with the understanding that a return favor will be granted.

j. *Lessen emotional dependency.* Don't sacredize family living. Don't put all your marbles in one jar. Engage in many enjoyable nonfamily activities and bring these experiences back to your family to share, rather than relying on your family group to provide you with entertainment.

k. *Avoid the red pencil mentality.* Focus more on what you like about one another rather than what you don't like. Stay away from flaw-finding that highlights personality blemishes.

l. *Actively solicit others' opinions.* Let others know you value their ideas by frequent "What do you think?" questions.

m. *Avoid the "Golden Rule."* Rather than assuming that others are just like you and believe "Do unto others as you would have them do unto you," allow for individual differences and abide by, "Do unto others as they would have you do unto them."

n. *Don't be too quick to advise.* Offer your resources with "Is there anything I can do to help?" Asking if help is wanted rather than tell what you think is needed. This is liable to win more friends and influence more people.

o. *Solicit others' help.* Rather than hint, whine, or scream for assistance, state "You are good at . . . , could you help me with this?" People often appreciate being called on to express themselves through their skills.

p. *Tease less, understand more.* Especially in times of hardship, bridging relationships can be better done by being supportive rather than taunting. When my (then) eight-year-old son learned that my first manuscript had been rejected, his comment was, "I'm sorry to hear your book didn't make it—especially since you are such a pro." Encouraging statements are likely to build more bridges and fewer walls than acrimonious comments.

q. *Disclose freely.* Spilling the beans about vital matters is one of the best ways to bond with another.

r. *Understand that fights pollute—not clear—the air.* A family that fights together is *less* likely to stay together. Realize that the supposed horrors of restraint are overplayed and that it is often best for your mental health and family living to not make an issue of your grievances.

s. *Distinguish quantity from quality.* Forcefully thinking that you "have to" spend time with your family will accomplish that goal. Deliberately explaining to yourself that you would "like to" will cause you to like it.

t. *See self and family interests as interlocking.* Promoting goodwill in the family rather than forcing your will on the family is a cornerstone of your happiness. Gently contributing to family well-being enhances your welfare. If your family is happier your life will be enriched because they will be more fun to be around.

u. *Approach problem solving unashamedly.* Openly admit and accept the fact that it is not a question of *if* your family has problems but what they are and what can realistically be done about them. If you mistakenly think you are a second-class citizen for having family problems, it will interfere with your ability to correct them.

Establishing perfectionistic rules about how family members "should," "must," "ought to," "are supposed to," "have got to" act toward one another runs counter to the fact that families are composed of imperfect people with differing opinions. In theory blood may seem thicker than water, but in reality people are different and differences often clash—if you let them. If you accept the truth that individual differences occur in the same family unit, peaceful coexistence can be established. From there, continue to see through the blood differences to promote family harmony and foster opportunities for more congenial relationships.

# Chapter 20

# Having a Sense of Humor in Proportion to What Ails You as a Parent

The following illustrations accentuate the value of humor to help get through parental hassles and responsibilities. Don't leave home or be in the home without it!

- When my two children were about nine and ten, they, my wife, and I toured the western part of the United States in an old 1972 Chevy van. Although in many ways we had the time of our lives, the long driving distances exacted a toll upon our patience and tolerance of one another's frustrating antics. To more quickly pass the driving time between distant cities we would play games such as "My father owns a grocery store," etc. My favorite was, "What would you do if Daddy dropped you off here?"
- When my daughter was about five years old she did something that violated my expectations of her. True to my fatherly responsibilities I corrected her, to which she responded, "Shut up!" I had read someplace that children were not to speak to their parents in this manner. Once I regrouped from the shock of her declaration I tried to back up and start all over again. I glared at her and very strongly inquired: "What did you say, young lady?" As usual she remained loyal to her direct approach of dealing with attempted intimidation and quickly and clearly shot back, "I said 'shut up'!" Dumbfounded, the only thing I could think of to say was, "That's what I thought you said," at which time we both began to laugh.
- When my daughter was four, she climbed up on my lap, looked at me with her beautiful, big brown eyes and asked,

"Daddy, if it takes two people to make one person, where did the first person come from?" I barely resisted the temptation to pass the buck and tell her to "go ask your mother" and instead took the time to discuss the varying theories on the matter. However, some years later she approached me while she was reading the book *Hotel*. She had come across two words that she failed to understand, and while pointing to them innocently inquired, "Daddy, what does sex orgy mean?" "Go ask your mother," I directed.

- On a Sunday afternoon my wife and I decided to slip into our bedroom for some privacy. My son Billy, who was eight years old at the time, could not resist trying to interrupt this luxury by gently knocking on the door and questioning, "Oh, Mom and Dad, you aren't doing anything in there that I wouldn't do are you?" I thought to myself, "I don't know; what wouldn't he do?"

When parents experience emotional disturbance in their parenting role, they are taking themselves and their relationship with their children too seriously. Enter humor. As seen in the previous examples, humor can cushion potentially awkward moments, reassert control, and help to provide a response without overreacting or personalizing the tides of parenthood. Humor helps you laugh so that you can take parent-child relationships in stride, without overdoing it, by exaggerating and escalating situations out of proportion. A sense of humor is a sense of perspective and proportion, which when established lends itself to better sharing your life with your child, without sacrificing your existence for your child. It enables you to stay involved with your child's life without getting entangled in it.

The goal of this chapter is to encourage laughter as a means of emotionally lightening up to better lubricate parent-child relationships. Laughter can help clear a path for the enlightenment that can occur when parents and children learn from each other. When something negative occurs in your parenting, laugh at yourself to ease your distress. Will Rogers said, "Everything is funny as long as it is happening to someone else." When something negative occurs in your parenting, laugh at yourself to ease your distress. If you learn how to find humor in your parenting role, it is unlikely that you will ever run out of comic material! Ethel Barrymore said, "You grow up after your first laugh–at yourself." Self-directed laughter can reduce heart/headaches that are unique to parenting when a child is likely to be more a bundle of responsibility than a bundle of joy. Some of the things our children do en route to maturity are difficult to make sense out of. A sense of humor can distract and provide emotional relief from such incongruities–all those things in parenting too numerous to mention that don't add up.

In addition to its distractionary, band-aid benefit, humor can also provide major surgery. Use it to not only feel better by experiencing that spun-out feeling we get in the back of our head when we laugh, but also to get better by finding humor within yourself as a parent. Such homemade humor can promote major changes in your philosophy of what it means to be a parent. A sense of humor adds proportion that can be both hopeful and helpful, light and enlightening. For instance, the following self-statements can lead to laughter *and* learning.

Laughter that *lightens:*

- "This too will pass–but does it have to take this long?"
- "Patience, crap; I'm going to kill him."
- "Things do seem to be getting worse at a slower rate."
- "Apparently when it comes to my children it's a matter of mind over matter; they don't mind and I don't matter."
- "Why oh why can't I have a low-maintenance child?"
- "You would think someone would hire my teenager while he still knows everything."
- "When I took on the job of being a parent I didn't realize that it would be like having a bowling alley installed in my head."
- "I take my kids everywhere–but why do they have to keep finding their way back home?"
- "If I can make my child miserable one more time I will have done my job."
- "What would this house be without my children? Quiet and paid-for would be my guess."
- "I thought parenting was supposed to be FUN!"
- "I'm at the end of my rope and I'm down to my last shred to hang on to."

- "When it comes to my parenting, I like things as they aren't."
- "My child told me he didn't ask to be born and I told him, 'That's right, and if you would have asked the answer would have been no!'"
- "I learned more about my child at his parent-teacher conference than I'd ever care to know."
- "My 18-year prison sentence to parenting seems to be going about as slow as molasses in January."

Laughter that *enlightens*–includes the following examples of parental humor that is both funny and educational:

- "I am not my parenting; I do my parenting. I am not holier-than-thou when my parenting succeeds, nor am I unworthier-than-all when my parenting fails."
- "I do not run the universe, therefore, I am not responsible for my children's problems and disturbances nor for discovering solutions to them."
- Which would be a more accurate statement to accept–"He should have learned his lessen by now," or "It would be better for me to accept that he hasn't learned by now and that there is a chance that he may never learn."
- "I can't sell my child a used car he doesn't want, so I will put away all my sales gimmicks."
- "If my child allegedly learns what he sees, why then isn't he a clone of me?"
- "My child is a basket case first and a family member second–an accident waiting to happen. Such wayward traits are facts of nature not nurture."
- "It's not true that only a percentage of children have emotional and/or behavioral problems–rather, eleven out of ten do. Why must my child not be among this elite group called humans?"
- "Better that I not play the rating game giving myself good or bad marks depending on how well my parenting is subsisting."
- "Many parenting problems are ego difficulties–problems of self-judgement–so an ego left on the doorstep prevents me from making myself emotionally dependent upon being a successful parent."

- "Better that I blend in with the flow of my child's attack rather than meet it head on."
- "The more my child gets the more she seems to want. Better that I not deprive her of the right to go without, thus circumventing this bottomless pit syndrome."
- "If I continue to bust a gut for the child I love because I can't muster up enough guts to use 'no' as a love word, I will likely end up despising the child that I have busted a gut for and failed to say 'no' to."
- "I am not an ass when my child and/or I act asininely."
- "If children learn what they see, I wish my child would take a closer look!"
- "How much is enough attention, praise, communication, understanding, or love without contributing to my child becoming an attention- love- understanding- and praise-seeking lush, slob, or junkie?"
- "Life is in part for lessons, and my child can learn both from my successes as well as from my blunders."
- "As far as I can tell, parents model two basic sets of knowledge–how to go through life in a sensible way and what potholes to avoid. Which set the child follows is to be determined by his free will."
- "If my love were the answer to everything or anything regarding my child's problems she would have many fewer difficulties; unfortunately the 'love conquers all fallacy' is just that."
- "I'll beat my child to the punch by laughing at myself. Laughing at myself feels better than his scorning me."

Parents are ill-prepared to manage the potholes, curve balls, and side-arm fast balls too numerous to mention that their children throw in their direction. When looking for light amusement and/or enlightenment regarding parenting concerns, either can be found within the boundaries of family experiences. Nothing is more interesting or funny than what goes on between people, especially those who live under the same roof. Owning up to rather than overlooking the human comedy has its advantages. In fact, humor itself is an (unfair) advantage. It is unfair that one person has the capacity to not take himself as seriously as someone else with opposing views.

When I was a young boy I would play basketball with my friend Richie Solberg. I had more basketball skill in my little finger than Richie had in his whole body. However, Richie had one unfair advantage over me. A split second before I was going to launch my jump shot he would yell loudly, "*Itchy balls* by Willie Scratchum." I found Richie's humor to be irresistible, would break out laughing, and of course miss my patented jump shot. It just wasn't fair that Richie could make up for his lack of athletic skill by simple humor.

Keeping your sense of humor as a parent is the equivalent to keeping your wits about you. It provides you with the advantage of tolerance since when you laugh at yourself you become more tolerant of yourself. Humor also promotes joy because laughter is a joyful experience. Without a sense of humor, parenting makes little sense at all. Perhaps more than any other advantage, humor provides a protective emotional coating, a psychological refuge that (a) can create a temporary distance between you and your children's oppositional antics, and (b) cushions the emotional blow when you find yourself in a circumstance involving your child that is far less than ideal. Such emotional relief in difficult times is nothing to sneeze at. Is humor the answer to everything, putting a damper on conflictual family interactions? Can it move mountains or perform miracles? The answer is no–although your child may often think that he can!

Like B'rer Rabbit who when surrounded by his larger captors, begged them, "Please, do whatever you want to do to me–except, don't throw me in the Briar Patch." For once paradoxical intention worked, and his captors disobeyed his command and threw him into the Briar Patch where he remained with all the amenities of life while safely protected from his enemies. So too, can humor protect you from your child's animosity. When at the end of your rope as a parent use humor to help you to hang on. By not taking your child as seriously as he is taking himself you are committing a kind, loving act. By taking a humorous step back rather than two somber steps forward, you contribute to dousing the flames of family conflict. Not that love and humor contain all the answers to parental problems, but combined they will likely contain a portion of the solution.

Chapter 21

# Questioning the Advisability
# of Unconditional Parental Love

"Unconditional" means just that–no strings attached. In the case of love, "unconditional" means "I'll love you no matter what you do in destructive ways toward me, yourself, others, or the niceties in life." The contention of this chapter is that if parents give the child such a blank check, parents may sign their life, peace, and quiet away to their offspring. Such a view goes beyond permissiveness to indulgence and is negative for all concerned. The child doesn't learn to earn and appreciate what he has; instead, he wrongly presumes that life is one big free lunch. The parents end up infinitely picking up after and trying to pacify their child, wearing their fingers to the bone on the offspring's behalf. The child expects others in the community–teachers, neighbors–to fill his bottomless pit with unconditional love. This "anything goes" and "I'll still love you with open arms" authorization gives the child a license to act as irresponsibly as he wishes, and in a sense rewards his demanding immaturity. Parents would do well to reclaim the bargaining power that they have relinquished in the name of "unconditional love." This is a term put forth to parents as being a sacred "must," i.e., "You must, under all conditions love your child unconditionally at all times, places, and circumstances. If you don't you are a sinister person for committing such a neglectful venial sin." Or so goes the declaration as it is attempted to be forced on the parents from the "love conquers all" experts.

Parents are human–not saints or angels. Let's face it, you would be saintly or angelic to continue to love someone who repeatedly and purposefully antagonizes and acts disrespectfully toward you, as some children will. Given such extreme parent-child conditions I submit it is appropriate for parents to fall out of love with their child while the child takes a second look at where his bread is buttered. There's no law that says you must keep loving someone who tries to tear your house apart. In fact, unless you put your best foot forward in a thunderous, unloving manner you are likely to continue to be taken advantage of.

This is not to say that you have to despise your child in order to discipline her. This would be the other extreme that would encourage overreaction as opposed to underreaction, or overdoing it as opposed to underdoing it. To have warm, loving feelings toward someone who is aggressively trying to take advantage of you makes it difficult to discourage such spiteful conduct. A more appropriate, no-nonsense, limit-setting approach is to put your love for your child on the back burner.

It's difficult to love a porcupine, and often it's more trouble than it's worth to try. Why deny the natural human response of not loving those who provide daily portions of hassle? Would it not be more honest, realistic, and emotionally healthier to give yourself permission to communicate to your child that your love is to be earned rather than given freely? What better way to prepare them for real life, where abundant, unearned love will not be provided? Others will love your child in accordance with his willingness to accommodate them, and not without an exchange of favors. So, why should you as parents believe it essential that you freely give of your love, with no anticipation of return? Show an interest in developing love for your child as you witness efforts on his or her part to better accommodate you. Expect rotation and balance as opposed to a one-sided "you for me and me for me" mentality. Doses of "feeling neutrality" that convey less dependence upon loving your child will likely increase interest and decrease "take for granted-ness" in the parent-child relationship.

When love is made to be conditional and provisional rather than unconditional, it yields more bargaining power in defense of your protection if not your sanity. Creating a temporary, and in some rare cases, permanent, emotional distance between you and your child may be just the remedy for parents who try too hard to do the impossible—gain their child's compliance by futility trying to transplant more helpful attitudes in his head and more satisfying feelings in his gut. Don't let yourself be taken advantage of by your child in the name of love. You do not need to become angry in order to set conditions in the parent-child relationship, nor should you feel guilty about your limit setting. In fact, refusing to give unconditional love to your child can paradoxically be one of the most *loving* things that you can do for him. This is so because such unloving attitudes are an honest reflection of the outside world–a "gut level" expression of honesty to self and child. This encourages your child to grow up by making it convenient for him to reassess the effects his lack of contributions to relationship upkeep have upon significant others in his social group. Love with no strings attached produces very minimal bargaining power, whereas calculated emotional neglect may increase child-management leverage.

So, if your unconditional love bucket has a hole in it and therefore is not working well, consider giving conditional love a try. When your child consistently displeases you by refusing to honor your household rules and values, consider giving conditional parental love a try. Admit that you are human enough not to love someone who continually sideswipes you behaviorally. Show that your love is not to be given freely, but is to be earned. Demonstrate this unashamedly and see if you can't fine-tune the procedure thereby gaining more effective child-rearing results. Eliminate the emotional disruption of guilt that comes from believing that you "should not," "must not" take such a rejective stance and that therefore you are a vile, wicked parent for courageously doing so. If you give your child an unconditional blank check it will likely result in emotional bankruptcy and you will resent it when your child takes you for granted. Conditional love will pay higher dividends in the long run in terms of your child's increased respect, compliance, and love. It is better to love someone enough to not let him or her take advantage of you. Discover for yourself if questioning the advisability of unconditional love doesn't turn out to be good advice.

# Chapter 22

# You Can Lead a Child to Water But You Can't Make Him Drink: Thirty-Four Guidelines for Effective and Efficient Parenting

It is difficult to teach things to people that they don't want to learn, and children often want to learn the opposite of what parents want to teach them. If a child is to learn a concept or skill he is required to be teachable, and to have inclinations toward learning. You will have your work cut out for you if you try to encourage a child to learn something he doesn't have a bias toward. "Bring up your children in the way they will become" is a suggestion that has a strong ring of truth to it. Human beings come into the world with strong tendencies to be the way they are—to go in the direction they are headed. After their first child, parents often take an environmental philosophy of parenting, seeing themselves as the primary molder of their child's personality. Following the birth of their second child, these same parents frequently begin to realize genetic influences in their child with likes and dislikes that are independent of their rearing methods. Children raised under the same family-values umbrella are often quite different. Children raised by adoptive parents will often exhibit similar eating habits and temperamental tendencies of their natural parents, whom they have never met!

For better or for worse, children possess preexisting leanings, and give vent to these tendencies in their family of record. Understanding and accepting these observations can be of value to parents in the following ways:

a. Encourages a sense of humility that comes from realizing the distinction between what you can and cannot do for and to your children.

b. Invites emotional relief stemming from convincing yourself that it is not what parents do to their children that is the problem—rather, it is what they fail to accept that they can't do for them, i.e., make them happy, change what has already happened, get them to take on values that would be better for them, reason them out of something they haven't been reasoned into. Such efforts in futility become like trying to sell the child a used car she doesn't want.

c. Knowing that they can't be all things to all children allows parents a better opportunity to share their lives with their child without sacrificing their lives for their child. Involvement can be maintained, but entanglement can be by-passed.

d. Conveniences self-acceptance. Most parental problems are problems of self-judgement and self-evaluation. If the child develops well the parent rates himself as "good." If the child encounters problems the parent views himself as "bad." This rating game can be avoided by appreciating that although parents *help* raise their child, there are aptitudes their offspring has that are givens—for no special reason.

e. Encourages the advantages that come from discouraging dependency on raising an emotionally healthy child. If parents are able to see themselves as enjoying people in their own right, they will feel less resentment when their child betrays their values. The less resentful they are, the more loving and capable they are likely to be.

f. Promotes a more well-rounded vision. By not putting all your eggs in the parental basket a broader view of life is allowed. Bringing such variety into your life makes you more fun to be around and less likely to dwell on what might not be working out in your parental role.

g. Discovery of general emotional unshackling. Providing self with an emotional breath of fresh air, lightening up rather than tightening up in the important area of parenting, allows a more free-wheeling, spirited approach to life generally. Accepting human limitations, applying self-acceptance principles, encouraging self-interest and self-reliance are all principles of emotional well-being that can be applied in and out of the parenting role.

Children use their differences with their parents as a convenient excuse to give vent to their remarkably fallible, problematic nature. Parents practically always turn out to be a disappointment in the eyes of their children—and if you don't believe me, ask your children! They typically insist that their parents be all things to all people—to take on all the favorable characteristics of all the other parents in the neighborhood. Regardless of how helpful a parent tries to be, the child will more often than not insist that the parent is trying to do him or her in. From a child's perspective, parents are often damned if they do, and damned if they don't. For example, a parent of a teenage boy who committed suicide sadly explained to me: "Whenever I would try to befriend him, he would tell me to leave him alone; when I would leave him alone, he would tell me, 'You don't love me.' " What's a parent to do! Read on.

Learning effective parenting skills is the substance of which most parent training programs are made. Effective parenting relates to using behavioral child management skills in an effort to make things right, gain compliance, and get the child to take on constructive values, i.e., getting things done rather than procrastinating, become more cooperative and less oppositional. Such teachings are all well and good. But what if your child is, as many seem to be, not very conditionable or reinforceable? Some children will swear by your rewards and some will swear at them. Behind every parenting storm cloud there isn't a silver lining, some are storm clouds through and through. Sometimes the solution to a parenting concern is to accept that there is no solution. I have been convinced for some time that as much as parents can use information on how to make things right, they can better use information on how to get themselves less upset when things go wrong. Enter efficient parenting.

Efficient parenting takes into account that as a parent you can do many of the "right" things in relating to your offspring and still get poor results. It takes into account what to do when your parenting role wavers and you seem to have run completely out of options. It recognizes that parenting is not all peaches and cream, not without its trials and tribulations. In addition to teaching what might make things right with and between you and your child, efficient parenting instructs how to get yourself less upset when things continue to go wrong. It incorporates some of the following ideas into its teachings:

- "I will do my best as a parent but I don't perfectionistically have to insist that I do the best."
- "Because my parenting role isn't going very well doesn't mean that the rest of my life has to come to a standstill."
- "I can run but I can't hide from my child's obvious limitations. Better that I accept these limits and not disadvantage my life because of them."
- "I don't have to put all my eggs in one parental basket; I can instead prove myself to be an enjoyable person in my own right."
- "Granted, watching my child falter is a helpless, sad, disappointing feeling. However, I am not required to amplify my regrets into hopelessness or disaster. What good would it do, and who would it benefit if I did?"
- "Due to his fallible nature and free will my child has a right to his limitations and the disadvantages they bring him."
- "Being a parent is an important job, but it is not all important or bigger than life."
- "I can use my parenting to work on my own mental health by not giving myself a report card with a bad mark when my parenting is going bad. My parenting is something I do, but it is not me; it may be going bad, but I'm not bad!"
- "Certainly I have invested a lot in my child's upbringing. However, there is no universal law that guarantees me a return on my investment. I need not take a woe-is-me, feel-sorry-for-myself attitude when my parental efforts do not pay dividends."
- "When it comes to community exposure of my child's problems I constitute a majority of one in stubbornly refusing to make myself feel ashamed about her problems. My child's behavior, like others' opinion, does not represent me."

- "I do not like, but I can tolerate the disappointments of parenthood. By not anguishing over them I put myself in a better position to do something about my concerns or to more gracefully accept what regretfully, cannot be changed."
- "Sometimes it's more what I don't do that is helpful. There is much value to caring less without becoming uncaring. It's easy to become a parent, but it takes a wise person to back away from matters of concern, to take a step back rather than two steps forward."

If you become less dependent on your parenting outcomes, you are less likely to take your child's contrary decisions personally. This will result in less hurt and anger, which in turn conveniences more love and clear-headed decision making. Rational, permissive ideas that allow you to cut yourself some emotional slack do not guarantee that you will make all the right decisions or that your choices will turn out right. However, they do better ensure that the state of mind with which you make your choices will be a thoughtful, all-things-considered one. After you establish parental efficiency by bringing yourself to a less dependent, more tolerant, self-accepting view, you will be more confident in picking and choosing from the following parental effectiveness skills in your efforts to better manage your child. Although not foolproof, these suggestions invite, encourage, and make convenient the prevention and resolution of parent-child conflicts.

1. *Reflective, active, attentive listening.* When in doubt, become an echo. Becoming an active sounding board of your child's feelings makes you hard to resist. Three little words, "I understand you," correctly applied can help take the wind out of your child's oppositional sails. Most communication between people involves the content, rather than the feeling, personal level. Responding to the who and not the what promotes building bridges instead of walls, conveniences others to gravitate toward you, thus becoming influenced more by you. Understanding how people feel rather than trying to talk them out of how they feel is one of the best standard operating procedures in cementing relationships. Attentively responding to your child's concerns or criticisms with "It

sounds like you really had a rough day at school"; "It seems like this is a hard decision for you"; or "I sense you don't like my house rules," rewards people for the openness of their positions, encouraging such direct communication in the future. The trick is not to say anything else. It's that something else, often in the form of unsolicited advice, that invites problems. Follow-up statements such as "It sounds like you really had a rough day at school. Why don't you study harder?"; "It seems like this is a difficult decision for you. Why don't you just do what I suggested?"; or "I sense you don't like my house rules. Why don't you check with your friends and see if theirs are any easier?" are all examples of not leaving well enough alone by doing active directing rather than active listening.

2. *Tell your child how you feel without telling her off.* Responsible self-expressional statements such as: "I have a problem with curfew violations and this is what I'm going to do about my problem: For each five minutes of curfew violation there will be thirty minutes subtracted from the regular curfew time for the next three nights"; "I make myself feel angry when the garbage isn't taken out"; or "I don't appreciate being talked to that way" are likely to gain your child's attention. Positions such as, "You make me angry when you don't cooperate, and if you don't knock it off you're never going to amount to anything" are likely to have the same effect as waving a red flag in front of a bull. "I" statements are more likely to gain attention and retention. "You" finger-pointing declarations will likely detain if not derail your intended message.

3. *Meeting halfway.* A willingness to bend without breaking can be helpful. Suggesting an option that may not be exactly what you want, or specifically what you child hoped for—but something in between these opposites—conveniences a workable compromise. Many a cold war has been thawed out with such neutralizing efforts, i.e., if your teenager wants a 2:00 a.m. curfew time and you want an 11:00 p.m. boundary, suggesting "How about 12:15 a.m.?" isn't going to guarantee the

matter will be resolved, but will invite a compromising climate on this and future issues.

4. *Better deal with your child's criticisms.* Children frequently act ungratefully. Understand that your child's criticisms do not represent you, but are annoyances to be responded rather than reacted to. Finding some truth to your child's worst criticisms may take the wind out of his contrary sails. For instance, if he accuses you of unfairness, or worse yet of being a lousy parent because you expect him to pick up his bedroom, don't fight fire with fire. Instead, understand that you're not on trial, answerable to your child; then, seek and report an element of truth in his accusation, i.e., "Maybe this isn't fair. You're right, *sometimes* I am a lousy parent . . . but I still expect you to pick up your room." Using your child's criticisms to work on increasing your tolerance softens a difficult situation.

5. *Constructive use of consequences.* Explain to your child what she can expect if she cooperates and what to expect if she doesn't. Then back off and let her decide what she is or isn't going to do. Presenting this fork in the road teaches her perhaps the most valuable lesson of all—how to make a decision. Offering her something positive to work toward for compliance and something negative to avoid in the event of noncompliance, forces her to make a decision. Even if she decides against your request and takes her medicine, she lives with the consequences of her choice. People often learn from the results of their choices and perhaps your child will too. Explain to your child that you want the garbage out by 4:00 p.m. For each five minutes after this time, if the garbage isn't taken out, she will have to go to bed 15 minutes earlier that night. This forces your child to decide under what conditions she wishes to spend her evening. Combining this negative to avoid with a positive to work toward, i.e., every evening that the garbage is taken out by 4:00 p.m. there will be a nighttime treat, provides a double-barreled approach to encouraging your child's motivation.

6. *Distinguish rights from privileges.* Regardless of how bad his or her conduct, a child has a right to food, clothing, and

shelter. Even people locked up for murder get that! However, extras such as Saturday afternoon matinees, trips to the ice cream parlor, biking, or car privileges can be placed under the heading of privileges to be earned. What was once a right can be turned into a privilege by parental decision. The elbow grease required to earn the privilege may cause it to be appreciated more.

7. *Use of Grandma's Rule.* Explain to the child that before he gets to do something he wants to do, i.e., go outside and play, he is required to do something he doesn't want to do, i.e., pick up his room or complete his homework. This can save a lot of wear and tear that comes from trying to convince a child to do something he doesn't want to do.

8. *Use of trade-offs.* "I'll scratch your back if you scratch mine" is a simple reality that can lubricate relationships. I'll agree to let you do this, i.e., use the car three times a week, if you agree to do that, i.e., clean your room every day. This is an example of how an exchange system can bring advantages to all concerned.

9. *Application of enormous detachment.* When your child is critical or complaining, to abruptly turn away from her or to remove yourself from her presence serves not only as a self-protective measure but discourages her future whinings. This disinterested procedure communicates that your relationship is to be earned and respected and that you do not intend to give with no expectation in return.

10. *Selective inattention.* An extension of the above method is to explain to your child that you are not willing to continue in a disagreement that is obviously going nowhere. Explain to him that you are willing to talk about other matters, but if he continues to expound on the issue you intend to remain silent. This prevents the escalation of differences of opinion.

11. *Don't take your child as seriously as she is taking herself.* Perhaps the most loving thing you can do for anyone is to not upset yourself because another is upset. Anytime there is one less person throwing gasoline on matters of concern, the smaller the fire is going to be, and the sooner others are likely

to settle down. Remaining concerned but not making yourself consumed will help to accomplish that.

12. *Tell your child more of what he can do, and less of what he can't.* It is important to instruct your child to avoid the risk factors in the world. However, an oversupply of "don't" tends to restrict the basis for the relationship. If you want to become more than a guardian to your child, put more emphasis on telling him what he *can* do. Don't wait for him to come to you and ask for a privilege, i.e., use the car, go to a movie. Seek him out and ask him if he would like to do so. Such an assertive show of interest is more likely to bring a show of appreciation.

13. *Ask more than tell.* A heavy dose of "you" questions, i.e., "What do you think?"; "What is your plan?"; or "If you were me, what would you do?" communicates that "What you say is important." Soliciting another's opinion is one of the best ways to make connections with that person.

14. *De-sacredize communication.* Don't pressure yourself to do alone what takes two to accomplish. Often, the more parents insist that they and their child communicate, the less conversation they are able to squeeze out of their child. The less you insist "We have to talk" and the more you believe "I would like to talk," the more naturally conversation is likely to flow. If your child sees that you will make yourself miserable if he doesn't communicate with you, he will use this as a bargaining chip in his efforts to control you.

15. *Lead with your values.* However, don't assume your child will become a clone of them. It would be silly to act like that as a human being you don't have bias as to what constitutes the good life. It would be equally silly to assume that just because you put your values on the table, that your child is going to buy into them—lock, stock, and barrel.

16. *Take on an "undamning acceptance" view of individual differences.* Respect for differences between you and your child temperamentally, socially, academically, religiously, lovingly, etc., prevents ill feelings between the two of you. Perhaps the best way to influence children is to accept them the way they are.

17. *View "no" as a love word.* "Never deprive a child of the right to go without." Parenting is not a popularity contest. Accepting this fact allows you to set limits on your child's requests. Setting boundaries for your child's behavior often will not be viewed by her as a show of caring, but that is beside the point in using your better judgement.

18. *Expect more of your child than he sometimes expects of himself.* Demonstrate a vote of confidence by consistently expecting your child to do better in projects that are within his potential, even when he tries to convince you and himself they are not.

19. *Don't overdo logic.* The main logic that many children follow is, "Be reasonable; see it my way." Anything short of such agreement is likely to fall on deaf ears. It is important to spell out your rules and consequences for violation of them; however, thinking that your children have to understand the rhyme and reason behind such realities is a different story. Your frustration will mount as you discover that no matter how well you explain the logic behind your decisions, it is not what your child wants to hear.

20. *Avoid excessive praise.* Too much of a good thing loses its benefit. To begin with, praise will not produce miracles in shaping your child's behavior. It is unlikely to be the answer to everything, and sometimes, to anything. Excessive praise can communicate to your child that gaining his compliance is all important. He then may use your desire for his cooperation as leverage against you. A moderate amount of praise for a child's performance is likely to encourage him to be less beholden to you and to have more of an impact on him when it is given. In addition, praise him simply for trying, not just for achievement.

21. *Modeling is helpful but not foolproof.* Display the virtues you wish your child to emulate, but as with praise, don't expect such efforts to work wonders. Children are likely to gravitate toward values that are a natural part of their temperament. When a teacher appears who models these values, the child will likely learn, however that person may not be you. Appreciating that by her nature a child tends to go in a particular

direction makes it easier for you to not pass judgement on yourself when your child has inevitable problems.

22. *Don't ask questions when you already know the answer.* This deceitful way of finding out whether your child will tell the truth only encourages the problem you are trying to discourage.

23. *Distinguish request from command.* If you want your child to do something, tell him you want it done. Don't ask if he will do it. If you ask him, you give him the option of refusing your request.

24. *Revoke privileges as discipline, but explain how they can be earned back.* Explain to your child that she has the power to change restriction by positive behavior. Take away privileges but tell her precisely what she has to do to earn them back, i.e., "Due to lateness I'm taking your bike away for one week; if you are home on time each night between now and then, you can have it back." This is opposed to "I'm taking your bike away for one month and no matter how often you're on time, you're not getting it back." The first declaration invites incentive, the second one encourages listlessness.

25. *Soften him up.* When addressing your child, use his first name, look him in the eyes, and touch him. Such action gets his attention and is an example of how little things, added up, can make a difference.

26. *Condense your message.* Limit yourself to eight to twelve words in your efforts to get your point across. Lecturing beyond that makes it tempting for your child to tune you out.

27. *Call to mind highlights.* Take a few minutes each day to focus on the concerns you *don't* have about your child. Such emphasis on the doughnut, rather than the hole in the doughnut, invites appreciation of and relief about your parenting role.

28. *Train others to think in positive ways about your child.* If you find others are focusing on your child's negative traits, prompt them to give you feedback about what they like about your child's behavior, i.e., at parent-teacher conferences, with others who supervise your child.

29. *Work on one correction at a time.* Try to do a lot of one thing

rather than a little of a lot of things in shaping your child's behavior. That way progress is likely to be more visible and everyone's efforts encouraged.

30. *Correction sooner, rather than later.* The best time to correct a bad habit is the first time it is seen. If you wait until after your child has slammed the door five times before you correct her, the habit will be more established and harder to break.

31. *Be specific in your correction.* Exactness in suggestion better paves the way for cooperation. "Pick your clothes up off the bedroom floor" is a clearer expectation than "shape up" or "be a good boy."

32. *Preferably state rules positively.* "Children who get their pajamas on now get a treat before bedtime" puts a more positive focus on this important part of the day than "If you don't put your pajamas on, you don't get a treat before bedtime."

33. *When possible, give him choices.* When decisions are negotiable, invite your child's opinion. Open-ended questions communicate that your child's input is important. People appreciate being asked their opinion about decisions that affect them. "What do you think would be fair?"; "What time can we expect you home?"; and "Would you like to use the car on Friday or Saturday night?" are examples of permitting your child to have some choices in his life.

34. *I saved the best for last: Practice a philosophy of enlightened self-interest in your parenting role.* Develop a philosophy of parenting that allows you to not concentrate solely on parenting. Instead, see yourself as an interesting person in your own right. Strive for a high-level solution to your concerns. Share your life with your child, but don't sacrifice yourself for your child. Find value in your own life. If your kids want to come along for the ride this is fine, but *not* necessary. In short, be self-interested. Put yourself first and your child a close second, rather than your child first and yourself a distant second. If you are less emotionally dependent on the outcome of your efforts as a parent, the less hurt and angry and the more loving, clearheaded, and consistent you are likely to

be. This is efficient parenting at its best—becoming less upset about your child's tendencies toward fallibility, accepting yourself in spite of them and moving on with your life regardless of parenting outcome.

Don't give your parenting responsibilities the limp hand. View the project of helping to raise your child as one of the most creative, important jobs you will take on in your lifetime—but not all important; a big part of your life, but not bigger than life. Invite, encourage, make it convenient for your child to do what is in his long-range best interest—but don't expect him or you to move mountains. Because you can't make *him* drink doesn't mean that *you* have to die of thirst. Parenting is one of the few jobs where you are successful if you work yourself *out* of a job. Fully appreciating that you have a life to live apart from being a parent is perhaps the most loving favor you can do for your child. Philosopher Eric Hoffer said, "Anyone can get on the train. It takes a wise person to know when to get off." Many can become a parent, but it takes a wise parent to know when to take a step back, rather than two steps forward in getting off the parental train. Provide your child with the water to drink, if not the food for thought. Do *your* best to present him with opportunities, while accepting that you can't do *the* best in guaranteeing him success.

Chapter 23

# The Ugly Duckling Syndrome:
# How to Duck Around
# and Over It

Humans naturally select against one another, especially when others are different. The more different other individuals are, the greater the tendency toward discrimination. This is standard operating procedure for interpersonal experiences. Most will be unconcerned about similarities while tending to dislike others' individual differences, except when it comes to family living. When one family member marches to a different drummer, that individual is often singled out as being unacceptable to the group. When determined to be too far away from the family norm, such personality and values deviation often becomes the target of harsh criticism. The different person is charged with being a psychological outcast, and given ugly treatment in accordance with such negative labeling. This chapter will review three facets of this distasteful syndrome: the purpose of such negative earmarking; typical faulty philosophies and coping mechanisms of the "duckling"; and recommendations the "ugly one" can use to experience a happier life in spite of his or her lack of family status.

1. Reasons behind the "ugly duckling" labeling:
   a. *Denial.* Fingerpointing in unison at one member permits other family members to conveniently deny their part in family troubles. Because it is not a question of *if* a family has problems, but rather *what* they are, denial via such ugly accusations can be made quickly accessible.
   b. *Excuse making.* Excusing one's negative conduct because

"I can't stand" the extreme manner of another member camouflages low frustration tolerance tendencies.

c.  *Personal insecurity.* Self-doubts can be pacified by channeling fears of one's own unusualness to someone else.

d.  *Rationalization.* Explaining away an individual's part in the family problematic plot can be accomplished by a version of "he makes me act this way" because of his ugly faults.

e.  *Comfort is derived from having a common enemy ("United we stand").* It is often emotionally uplifting to look down on someone else. When that someone else is so different from you and under the same roof besides, emotional relief is close at hand.

f.  *Human defensiveness.* When humans think they have to explain or defend their wrongdoings they will avoid putting themselves on trial by blaming a family bystander. Often this is the one who is the most obviously different.

g.  *Self-definitions.* When an individual thinks he is required to define himself by his bad mistakes, he will often execute a complete turnaround, and rather than blame himself will instead scapegoat another family member.

h.  *Regulates conflicts and disagreements and keeps the families stress level down.* If conflicts and disagreements can focus on one unit member, conflicts are channeled and free-for-all arguments are avoided. This can provide the majority of members with a minimum of stress between them because their negative feelings are routed to the black sheep of the group.

i.  *Long-standing unwantedness or unwanted differences.* If a member was born into the world at the wrong time, in the wrong place, with the wrong character traits and disposition that go against the grain of family tradition, her chances of gaining her family's acceptance may be nil. Some examples of extreme negative family selection are:

• The young adult man who told me that his father, who was a farmer, often told him, "I should have raised a pig. I would have gotten more profit."

- The now older man who was taunted by his family because he was schooled in special education classes while his siblings were honor roll students.
- The 19-year-old lady who explained to me that her mother, for whatever reason, never really liked her. This was most obvious when at age 17 she informed her mother that she had just overdosed on drugs, and her mother simply turned around and went out for the evening as originally planned.
- A mother who told me that for years she secretly harbored hatred for her son because he looked so much like his absentee father.
- A young man who now hated his mother because she would demonstrate her spite for him by sending him to school dressed partially as a female.
- A father who would consistently yell at his attention deficit disorder son, "I hate you. I wish you were dead!"
- A family with a history of producing males to carry on the "_____ and sons" family business, but at the end of the mother's child-bearing years had but one daughter who was designated to serve as this family's scapegoat.
- A father whose son had not measured up in terms of expected achievement told his son to legally change his last name.

2. Normal but not healthy methods of coping by the "Ugly Duckling": Because of the general human tendency to judge oneself by others' approval or lack of it, and due to our cultural belief that if your family thinks badly of you, you're bad and worthless, a large majority of the "Ugly Duckling" population believe that they must walk around for the rest of their lives with their head hanging between their legs. Figuratively and sometimes literally having a face that not even a mother could love is often seen as reason to go through life as a second-class citizen. Self-acceptance, even in the face of outright discrimination from significant others seems an impossible dream to the earmarked one. When at the bottom of the family pecking order, the human tendency is to define oneself by one's low family ranking. Self-depreciation occurs by con-

cluding that there must be something drastically wrong with you if your own family members turn their back on you. Abuse of alcohol and other drugs, failure to set constructive goals that are in contrast to a view of oneself as a failure, choosing a partner that substantiates your "loser" image, choosing associates who like you are down on themselves, participating in perfectionistic methods of proving self, engaging in risk-taking stunts that leave your social group in awe are all examples of self-defeating methods of coping with the "Ugly Duckling" designation.

3. Recommendations for overcoming the image of low person on the family totem pole:

a. *Make the distinction between being dealt a bad hand in life and playing a bad hand well.* Encourage yourself and teach others that you can reshuffle the hand nature and nurture dealt you and have the freedom to deal yourself a better hand.

b. *Constructive use of attribution.* What does your family members' harsh assessment of you tell you about them? Try to realize that their malice toward you does not represent you, but rather their own ignorance, problems, and disturbance. Then,

c. *Don't evaluate yourself by their deficiencies.* Avoid estimating, defining, and/or rating yourself by others ill-advised judgements. Convince yourself that other family members' opinions do *not* equal you.

d. *See that your family doesn't disturb you.* However, you can disturb yourself about your family–if you allow it. Whether you be termed the "family scapegoat" "identified patient," "symptom bearer," or some other fancy label used by those who describe what goes on in family systems, you can use your capacity for emotional self-sufficiency to not disturb yourself by such psychological trashings.

e. *Understand that being influenced and affected by your family is light years apart from disturbing yourself about them.* Because of your preference for kinder and gentler treatment, you are naturally not going to be an emotional island when treated in displeasing ways by your family. However, by not overreacting to and personalizing such discrimination you can better regulate your feelings, remaining dissatisfied and disappointed by their antics without angrily or hurtfully disturbing yourself. Try to remember what George Bernard Shaw said, "Things don't happen to me–I happen to them."

f. *Opt for nonpresumptuousness.* Don't presume the emotional worst, otherwise you give yourself a heavy dose of the self-fulfilling promise. People tend to act the way they see themselves. If you presume a catastrophic outcome from others' negative labeling you may bring it about. Consider the option of emotional containment before serving yourself the inevitability of emotional defeat.

g. *Appreciate that it has been done before.* Many others have overcome the wiles of family scapegoating to establish a fulfilling life of their own–sometimes *because* of their shoddy upbringing. To quote Charles Dickens: "You can learn manners from those who have none."

h. *Challenge yourself to unblock yourself from suggestibility, gullibility, and normalcy.* Our culture anticipates that individuals will suffer emotional disturbance in the event of family discrimination. In fact, individuals are often told they are in denial if they conclude that they are *not* emotionally ruptured due to a lifelong exposure to disturbed family members. For instance, being associated with an alcoholic does not cause irreparable emotional harm as the codependent zealots would like to lead us to believe. It is *not* terrible to be an adult child of an alcoholic parent and *not* suffer emotional torment. Emotional disturbance can be challenged by refusing to personalize and overreact to family members' problems and frustrations. One can determine for him or herself whether to give blind adherence to the cultural suggestion that the emotional worst will always occur given certain family criticisms against one of its members.

i. Realize that others outside your family will vote for you for the same reason those in the family will impeach you.

Others' opinions of you are a reflection of their tastes and preferences. Try to give more thought to others' favorable impressions—even when they occur outside your family of origin.

Living with people who disparage you is an ugly experience. However, it need not be a foregone conclusion that your life must come to a screeching halt because of such a dastardly lack of accommodation. Instead, you can duck the verbal punches and at the same time work around and over tendencies to personalize and overreact to such scenes. Views that favor the use of logic and reason in the service of one's emotions will have you creating your own, more pleasant life picture.

Chapter 24

# When Baby Makes Three: Children As Intrusion

Putting it mildly, children can be highly inconvenient. Putting it moderately, two is company, three is a crowd. Putting it strongly and to quote W. C. Fields, "Anyone who hates children and dogs can't be all bad." All parents can identify with these three degrees of experience. The onset of children definitely brings a dimension to family living that includes many unexpected occurrences if not shocks, oftentimes more than the would-be parents bargained for. Unless a plan is developed, preferably prior to the child's arrival, regarding what to expect in lifestyle adjustments, high frustration at best and chaos at worst are likely to occur. This chapter is not an attempt to tell prospective parents exactly what is going to happen in the post-birth or adoption era. Rather it is to encourage them to begin to realize complications can arise when the stork makes an appearance. An ounce of prevention is worth all the cure that can be mustered in coping with the onset of parenting.

Adjustments, tolerance, and acceptance are necessary to avoid disorganization. The following list discusses dimensions to family living that are affected when baby makes three.

1. *Financial adjustments.* Three can live as cheaply as two–if at least one doesn't eat. Children cost money and represent a poor financial investment. Without financial planning with foresight parents can end up in the poorhouse between everyday spending on the basics and other more isolated expenses such as dental work, car insurance, legal expenses, and career education. Monetary adjustments include all the things that parents will be required to cut back on, if not go without, such

as buying a later model car, eating out, and newer furniture following the onset of child rearing.

2. *Career adjustments.* Due to parental responsibilities and the wish to be more closely involved with their child, educational and career goals are often put on hold. Often it appears that there is not enough time in the day to balance work with parental ambitions.

3. *Time together is at a premium.* Couples used to immediate, direct accessibility to one another now have a competitor for their time with one another. No longer is it convenient to quickly determine to have lunch together or to see a movie on their afternoons or evenings off work. Baby-sitting, breast feeding, and the child's eating and sleeping schedule must now be given consideration. This causes couples to remark to themselves, "It ain't as simple as it used to be, dear."

4. *More frequent in-law/relative involvement.* For better or for worse, a couple with children is more likely to get more visits from relatives. Sometimes these visits are planned, and sometimes they are of the "drop by when it is inconvenient" variety. These visitations, however well meaning they might be, further tighten the parents' complicated schedule.

5. *Finding time for old friends*—especially those without children—who persist in seeking your companionship to the frequency it was B.C. (Before Children), becomes harder to arrange. Sometimes these associates will be offended by your inaccessibility due to parent-child commitments. They don't seem to understand that with a new life comes a different life with a new schedule.

6. *There is less time for hobbies and special projects.* What was once a weekend or after-work passion becomes a dimly lit interest that you are now having a hard time devoting attention to.

7. *Time for solitary endeavors becomes a luxury.* That bike ride through the countryside, the jog by the lake, reading, or just plain thinking time becomes as difficult as squeezing juice out of a turnip. You just don't seem to be able to find the time for yourself that you used to.

8. *Vacations, gardening, and other recreational items must also take a back seat.* Camping, long trips, and recreational tournaments of yesteryears become nonexistent in favor of the new arrival.

What is a mother–and father–to do? What can be done to squeeze more happiness out of a new lifestyle so that it can be seen as different but not overly troublesome? The following suggestions are made so that parents can prepare for their lifestyle adjustments while giving themselves some emotional slack in doing so–running these intrusive elements instead of the intrusions running them.

1. *Appreciate the temporary nature of parenthood.* Consistently remind yourself that "This is not going to last forever. This too will end." This hope that can get you through the nights ahead is the purpose of this perspective.
2. *Briefly look back to and appreciate the fond memories of the carefree days gone by.* Then–
3. Look ahead to the time these days return and appreciate that life will eventually come full circle. When you have that basis for comparison, you will likely appreciate life more.
4. *Choose special times.* True, you will be unable to be as free as before the arrival of your child, but that doesn't mean you can't recapture some of the "without children" benefits. Look for mini opportunities to enjoy what you once did on a larger scale.
5. *Consistently be on the lookout for temporary, substitute caregivers.* Exchange child care favors with friends, ask relatives to take care of your child–sometimes for days at a time. This type of extended respite can help to recharge your batteries for tolerance and patience.
6. *Don't feel guilty or ashamed for taking extended time-outs or for feeling resentment toward your child when you are unable to be less confined by him.* Time away will help you to be a more effective and efficient parent. It is unlikely that you will be the one set of parents who hasn't harbored bitter feelings toward their child. Try to dissolve this anger, but don't put yourself down for having it. After all, compassion often begins at home and if you are able to inject it in yourself, the

better able you will be to give it to your child when he or she exhibits trying behaviors.

7. *Avoid all-or-nothing thinking.* Stay away from notions that imply all parenting and no play. Such ideas make parenting a dull project. You are not required to put your enjoyments and ambitions totally on ice. Granted, parenting has more of its share of limitations in thwarting personal ambitions. However, these limitations can be worked out sometimes so that you can explore individual goals while still devoting adequate attention to your parental responsibilities.

8. *Talk to other parents in similar predicaments.* In addition to the advantage of emotional support brainstorming to examine how others cope with juggling their parenting role with other demands, can produce problem-solving ideas.

9. *Try to develop a philosophy of enlightened self-interest.* Establish a distinction between putting yourself first and your child a close second rather than your child first and yourself a distant second. This will prevent simply waiting for your child to grow away from you before you can invest time, money, and other advantages to and in yourself.

10. *Adopt a philosophy of give and take, rotation and balance rather than giving your child undivided time and attention.* Too much devotion to your child not only spoils the child but leads you to resent both yourself and the child—he for being spoiled rotten and you for letting it happen.

Hang on to your hats, potential parents! Your life may never be the same in this post-child era! Don't expect the kind of personal freedom that you had to continue after children burst into your life. Realizing this will put you in a better position to cushion the inconvenience that goes along with bringing a child into the world. You may never learn to savor these almost constant intrusions, but perhaps you will be able to cope with them. With tolerance and acceptance in place, you will be in a better position to experience more of the perks that go along with the present company of three.

Chapter 25

# The Ultimate Childhood Daydream: Being Able to Order Parents on a Silver Platter

When it comes to evaluating their parents, most children insist that peaches are not enough, but that they want pears, plums, and all the other fruits (of their parents' labor) besides. This fruity idea is seen in their commanding message and tone that reflects the insistence that they be the one child in the universe who has perfect parents. This fairy-tale command can have you backpeddling, over-explaining yourself while putting yourself in an exceedingly defensive posture as a parent. This chapter is to assist parents to emotionally liberate themselves so as not get caught up in their children's hazy, silver-platter belief. Parents are not on trial, answerable to their child when they commit human blunders. If they think that they are accountable to their child's complaints and therefore "must" get the child to understand and accept their directives and opinions, they will likely end up working for the child's demands and trying to fulfill never-ending requests.

This view includes the notion that parents are required to acquire all the favorable traits and characteristics of other parents in the family's neighborhood and beyond. They are to be all things to their children, all of the time, and seemingly the child will not settle for anything less. If the parents go for such perfectionistic bait, they will not only find an impossible mandate on their hands, but also an impossible-acting child. This child will not run out of unrealistic expectations, demanding that the silver-platter expectations be made a reality. Though fulfillment of this fantasy lies somewhere beyond a pot of gold at the end of a rainbow, the child will likely be the last to understand and accept the fact that he has an imperfect parent in an imperfect world. The child would do equally as well to write a letter to Santa Claus requesting an ideal parent rather than voice this command to parents.

Often the closer one gets to a goal, the more tarnished it becomes. In the absence of a basis for comparison children will vote for an alternative that is different from everyday reality for them, i.e., glorifying what it would be like to live with their friends' parents, with a relative, in a foster home, or even on their own. My experience has been that many children who either run away from home or who live in a foster home or other out of home placement for a time begin to realize that often the grass isn't greener on the other side of the fence. So, when your child demands that you reorder your values to suit him or else he will ship out, chalk it up to childhood (in)experience. Don't take it personally. Don't depreciate yourself while in the teeth of your child's insistences that you revoke your personality and general way of doing business with your world. Instead, invoke your own self-acceptance, don't give yourself bad marks as a parent due to your child's badly distorted, unrealistic thinking. The child may be too immature to appreciate the reality that you, like all humans, have a right to be wrong. Children often arrive at their view of parents with the following distorted perspectives:

- "My parents should be more like other parents."
- "Why can't my parents let me do what other kids' parents let them do?"
- "My parents are too old-fashioned compared to other parents I know."
- "My parents' house rules and punishments are stricter and harder than those of other parents."
- "I could be a lot happier living someplace else."
- "My parents try to make me unhappy on purpose and they have succeeded!"
- "I deserve better parents."
- "Because I didn't ask to be born, I should now be able to make all of my own choices."
- "My parents are never fair."

- "Every time I ask my parents if I can do something, they say no."
- "My parents always disagree with me."
- "My parents never understand me."
- "My parents never agree with me."
- "If they are not going to let me do what I want to do, they should let me live somewhere else."

Parental perspectives that take pressure off by countering the child's perfectionistic insistences include:

- "I'll chalk it up to my child's lack of a broader vision."
- "If I didn't have a basis for comparison, I might think that way too."
- "When I was that age I may have thought the same way."
- "He's only trying to find his separate identity."
- "I need not take this personally. My child's demands do not equal me."
- "I can't be all things to all people and I'm not going to even try."
- "I need not go for my child's demanding bait."
- "I am not beholden to get my child to exaggerate less."
- "Because my child pours it on so thick with her complaints, I need not compound such exaggerations."
- "Love and agreement or permissions often don't go hand in hand, but it is up to my child to learn that. I can't teach him, and the more I try to do his thinking for him the more I will be likely to further muddy the waters between us."
- "Perhaps one day my child will realize that I'm not such a bad parent. In the meantime, I'll patiently wait her out."
- "As my child is exposed to more of life's harsh realities he will be more likely to conclude that not only is his home where his head and heart are, but also where his bread is buttered. Let me concentrate more on pursuing my own happiness while hoping that time will come sooner rather than later."

Your child, like all humans, can run but cannot hide; may be able to temporarily escape in action/and or in fantasy from what he finds unacceptable in life generally and in his parents specifically. Until that long and eagerly awaited day arrives when he begins to see through his foggy daydream, depend more on yourself and less on your relationship with him. Take on a philosophy of enlightened parental self-interest whereby you put yourself first and his demands for you second, thus you won't turn his daydream into your nightmare and end up resenting your Herculean, but impossible, efforts to fulfill his ideal parental fantasies.

# Chapter 26

# When It's Good
# to Set a Bad Example:
# Learning Manners
# from Those Who Have Few

Just as one can learn honesty from those who steal from them, so too, as Charles Dickens said, "You can learn manners from those who have few"—*if* you play your cards right. That is a big *if* because ordinarily humans don't take very kindly to getting the short end of the stick in practically any circumstance. This is especially so in family relationships where children and adult children will typically hoot and howl, moan and groan when they discover that they weren't the one person in the universe born of perfect parents in a perfect family. Such insight, when accepted rather than protested against, can be used to one's advantage. Parents, from my observation, demonstrate matters and manners of life that fall under the umbrella of two general categories:

1. How to go through life in a sensible way that contributes to long-range happiness and survival. Examples of such favorable presentations include:
   - Minimize impatience and demandingness.
   - Have a decent respect for individual differences.
   - Accept others', as well as your right to be wrong.
   - Set long-range goals even if it requires you to make short-run sacrifices.
   - Wisely regulate your relationship with food and alcohol.

- To not take others' opinions personally.
- Prepare for some sort of vocation en route to being self-supporting.
- Encourage independent decision making.
- Do unto others as *they* would have you do unto them.
- Emphasize the value of kindness, understanding, and encouragement.
- Stay one step ahead of paying your bills.
- Value and nourish the bonding relationships one chooses to become a part of.
- Appreciate the value of being friendly and to have friends.

2. How "not to do it" by avoiding those actions that you have witnessed in your parents conduct that will work against your best interests, such as:
   - Figuratively putting your foot in your mouth by speaking without prior thought.
   - Finding the personality blemishes in others and then focusing on them.
   - Lying and deceitfulness.
   - Perpetrating physical, verbal, and/or sexual abuse.
   - Neglect of loved ones.
   - Spending without thought for what tomorrow will bring in terms of your ability to pay back.
   - Overindulging in alcohol and other drugs.
   - Engaging in outright criminal and other antisocial behavior.
   - Making virtually no effort to understand others.
   - Demanding that one has his or her own way.
   - Approaching life in a procrastinating, helter-skelter way.

From these two separate smorgasbords of behaviors, some obviously of long-range value, and some not, the child can then pick and choose those conducts that he wishes to continue to use. With free will in force the child eventually will be stripped of any legitimate reason to cop out—he can choose to keep alive or discard any of the behavioral offerings presented as well as those he develops himself. He can see that if he is/were told and/or taught these same self-defeating manners, messages, and behaviors today, he would not be required to carry them forward simply because he was encouraged or instructed to.

Why and when, though, can it be good to be exposed to a bad example? Ironies and paradoxes of life frequently don't add up until you search for the subtle, hidden truth behind them. Ironical ideas (a) seem contradictory, (b) drive home a message, and (c) imply an alternative if you read between the lines. The ideas of when it's good to be set upon by a bad example and then learning manners from those who have few reflects these three ingredients. It can be good to be exposed to bad examples because:

1. *It can prevent culture shock that occurs when it is discovered that the rest of the world doesn't display the kind manners that your parents did.* This abrupt splash of cold water in your face usually occurs at the onset of school. If your parents bent over backwards to expose you to their good manners, when you hit the streets of reality a bad, rude awakening is likely to occur. Not that the child won't survive such a contrast between the polite cushion that she has become accustomed to, but some difficult reality adjustments are likely to be in order. On the other hand, bad examples of whatever sort you have experienced can expedite a smoother transition to life outside the psychological womb.

2. *Such poor actions in significant others provide unlimited opportunity for learning*—but we are back to that *if* you play your cards right. The more graphic and dramatic the "how not to do it" examples are, the more potential there is for learning. Thinking back on the most gruesome experiences one has had often produces the most enduring learnings.

3. *It can allow for a fuller appreciation of the remarkable fallibility of human beings.* Seeing firsthand humans' flawed nature can help detract from perfectionistic tendencies toward self, others, and life. In that happiness is a direct ratio between what you expect and what you get, bad experiences can encourage you to expect less, consequently permitting you to squeeze more happiness out of life.

4. *It borrows from the idea that children often want to learn the opposite of what parents wish to teach them.* As a result of

their oppositional nature, if parents inadvertently or purpose-fully attempt to transmit bad habits to their children they may just as well as not send themselves in a "good" direction.

5. *Not only is the child more likely to learn better from the school of hard knocks stemming from bad examples*—but because of the negative impact, he is more likely to remember his lessons longer.

6. *It allows for more personality versatility related to the direct experiences of the bittersweet nature of life.* Life can be like sucking honey from a thorn, often the sooner one can get acclimated to this good in bad and bad in good rotation and balance, the better.

7. *Encourages a deterrent for in the future.* For instance, if you have been abused as a child, recalling your distain for such unfortunate occurrences can help head off any inclinations you might have to repeat history with your own children.

The message of this chapter is that you can use earlier adversity to improve the quality of your life. By being wise enough not to repeat others' mistakes, otherwise negative outcomes can be avoided. Firsthand exposure to bad manners can lead to a better assurance of a happier existence. Use adversity to work for you; welcome it as an opportunity to point yourself in a more fruitful direction. Reshuffle the cards and deal yourself a better hand that gives you more resources to allow you to enhance, rather than handicap, the momentum of your life. See that you control more of the variables of and the options to your future than you once did. Learn how to set your own good example by finding the good that lies in the opposite of what was originally bad.

# Chapter 27

# Parenting Is a Nice Place to Visit, but Inadvisable to Stay: Working Yourself Out of a Job While Retaining Its Joys

Being a parent can be one of the biggest challenges, and most creative experiences in one's life cycle. However, like most interpersonal highlights it is important not to wear out your welcome, and to instead get out when the getting is good. The timing for parents and children moving on with their lives and out from one another is a judgment call for which there are no pat answers, only guidelines. The time for moving on and out comes for practically everyone. For some it comes at midnight on the child's eighteenth birthday; for others it might not be until on or around the parents' twenty-fifth wedding anniversary. This chapter will present some guidelines for good and bad reasons for letting go of the practicalities of parent-child relationships. It is sufficient to say that parents and children getting out of each others' hair is a healthy eventuality for most all concerned from a practical as well as an emotionally dependent standpoint.

Parenting is one of those rare tasks that when successful, you find yourself without work. To linger as a parent or child is to invite unhealthy dependence and mutual resentment. Yet, one can leave the nest for good and bad reasons; to break the umbilical cord is good, to rip it isn't so good. It is not so much when this developmental task of parting is accomplished but the reasons one gives oneself for doing so. Reasons that reflect demands and exaggerate life's philosophies in either/both parent and/or child are best avoided in favor of those that reflect preference and emotional containment. The self-sentences in Table 27.1 and Table 27.2 reflect rigid vs. flexible thinking on the part of both parent and child while attempting to sever long-lasting dependency.

Parenting truly can be a nice place to visit, but its uniqueness does not necessarily qualify it as a nice place to stay. When is it time to lessen parent-child involvement? When is it time not to escalate emotional entanglement by doing things for the child that the child can do for him or herself?

The following advice signals parents and children that the job of the former is over, that the parent can take a back seat and enjoy observing the child's budding self-reliance. Realizing that the job is over, that what can be done has been done or at least tried, can pave the way to experiencing the joys of associating with the finished product. Pressure is taken off both parents and children when they experience the relief of an interdependent relationship. The warning signals of fused parent-child relationships referred to above are when:

a. *"Take for grantedness" is allowed to set in.* If it is presumed that business as usual will continue with no light at the end of the tunnel, it may be time to propose more long-term possibilities for an eventual departure.

b. *Lack of enlightened self-parent interest.* Whereby the parent ends up consistently doing things for the child that the child can do for himself.

c. *Evidence of the Bottomless Pit syndrome.* Dependency has been allowed to go too far when the parent makes ongoing provisions that do not exhaust the childs wishes, wants, and desires.

d. *Ungratefulness is openly expressed.* Ingratitude goes beyond take for grantedness in that it incorporates open complaints from the child who considers it her birthright to "have it all."

e. *Lack of rotation and balance becomes a dominating force.* You for me and me for me is the motto of the child who has been allowed to stick around too long rather than fend for himself.

f. *No preparation given for severance (without pay).* When the child is allowed to drift from job to job, school to school, or do whatever her heart desires, the time is to eliminate such

TABLE 27.1

| Irrational and Inadvisable Reasons/ Ideas for Parents to Bolt Parenthood | Rational Advisable Counters Relating to the Parenting Role |
| --- | --- |
| 1. "I can't stand a minute more of my child's friskiness." | "Though tolerable, I choose not to continue to expose myself to such ingratitude. Such ongoing permissiveness doesn't encourage my child to grow up and makes it convenient for me to feel resentful toward him." |
| 2. "She continues to act just as bad as her mother/father (absentee or emotionally divorced parent). She is bad for doing so and she can get get out of here as fast as her legs can carry her." | "Though there is more than a slight resemblance to her father/mother, these bad traits do not mean my child is bad. Now, do I want her to leave or offer that she stay providing certain preexisting conditions are modified?" |
| 3. "I've been forced to put up with and be held accountable for all his problems of the past eighteen years and absolutely no second chances will be given—not under any different conditions whatsoever." | "True, I have been left holding the bag in many of my child's problematic occasions, but now that he is eighteen and legally responsible for herself perhaps he will show greater accountability for himself. Let me decide whether to opt for giving him the opportunity for a new beginning." |
| 4. "I absolutely must let go of helping out in my child's life because if I don't, others will disapprove and think I'm babying her—and such social misgivings would be horrible." | "When and if the time comes that I believe it to be in my child's and my best interests to do so, I will take action because I, more than anyone else, will know when to do so." |
| 5. "No one else that I know hangs on as long as I do as a parent and it is wrong for me not to use others as a barometer for my decision." | "One size doesn't fit all. I'll use my own judgment as a barometer of what is best for me." |

TABLE 27.2

| Irrational and Inadvisable Reasons/Ideas for Children to Leave Home | Rational, Advisable Counters/Reasons for Children to Leave Home |
|---|---|
| 1. "I NEED my total independence come hell or high water, and I must move out in order to achieve it." | "Emotional independence is a state of mind and something that I can achieve whether I stay or leave the nest." |
| 2. "I absolutely must prove my ability to care for myself." | "I have nothing to prove. Now do I want or do I not want to move out?" |
| 3. "Practically all individuals in my social group are now living on their own and reminding me that I'm not. I must quell their criticisms by moving out myself." | "True, practically all my friends no longer live with their parents; false, that I must be just like them rather than the individual (who can think for myself) that I am." |
| 4. "I've been taunting my parents for many years about my intentions to break away from them the split second that I reach legal age; therefore I must not reconsider any other alternatives at this time." | "True that I've been flaunting my independence in power struggles with my parents for years; but just because my independent opportunity is upon me doesn't mean that I can't reconsider based on the present realities that beset me." |
| 5. "There is an absolute cut-off point beyond which no one should ever remain dependent on a parent." | "All people and circumstances are different and there is no universal yardstick by which to measure the day of independent reckoning." |

inconsistent, fickle, immature conduct, with the words "do, don't drift."

g. *Lack of listening.* When an overabundance of unsolicited advice from the parent usually always falls on deaf ears it may well be time for the parent to point to the door unless the offspring agrees to take suggestions, which are often a reflection of house rules.

h. *Flaunting of homestead expectations.* An "anything goes" philosophy often ends up with "nothing goes" right. Until people learn to know and trust what to expect in one another, they may be better off living apart.

i. *When parents find themselves ready for take off in their second life as civilian nonparents.* Having willfully completed the moral obligations of their parenting role, parents often look forward to life beyond parenting in the form of a second career, further education/training in their present career, a long-dreamed-about hobby or other vital absorption. To hold back from such significant hopes and dreams is to invite resentment; to move forward with new ideals is to invite contentment.

j. *An unwillingness or inability to compromise.* When unable to consistently bend without breaking when at loggerheads, consideration of a mutually agreed-upon separation may be in order, before the relationship totally disintegrates.

k. *A conscious, healthy desire on the part of all parties concerned to spread their wings.* Moving away from one another does not need to happen in a cloud of dust. It can be done in civilized, well-planned, appreciative ways, with consideration for difficult times. Moving out does not have to be all push and broom, hardship and resentment. Instead, it can be done in a spirit of cooperation and collaboration whereby individuals change jobs in an amicable manner thus retaining the joys from the work completed.

Live a little, love a little, give a little, and take a little. Especially take the learnings and goodwill from, and future anticipations for, you and your child. Eric Hoffer said, "Anyone can get on the train. It takes a wise person to know when to get off." Practically anyone can become a parent; it takes wise parents to know when to get off the parental train and to get on with the rest of their lives.

Chapter 28

# Haven on Earth:
# Protecting Yourself from
# the Oppositional-Acting Child

Parents who have spent a rainy Sunday afternoon with their child, or perhaps even a clear and sunny Sunday afternoon with their child, will usually admit that children are more buckets of responsibility than they are bundles of joy. In the long haul, children are more likely to badger, hassle, and banter with their parents than they are to comfort, soothe, or delight them. Unless the parent creates a refuge from these negative realities of parenting, resentment and helplessness will likely set in. If annoyances are not contained due to the parents' inability to smooth out their child's frustrating behavior, or at least protect themselves from it, a hell rather than a haven on earth is likely to occur.

Distancing yourself from your child's unmannerly ways involves being both emotional and practical, philosophic and pragmatic. These two aspects of haven building, emotional and behavioral, will be reviewed in this chapter.

## EMOTIONAL, PHILOSOPHIC,
## AND INNER INSULATION

To protect your emotions from the opposition try to use reason and logic. Do this in an orderly fashion by not putting the cart before the horse. Rid yourself of emotional interferences first, by getting yourself less upset about your child's oppositionalism. Then use the protective expressions and behavioral shields described in the section on behavioral insulation (p. 201). Realize that it is not your child's conduct that disturbs you and causes you to feel angry, hurt, guilty, or enraged, but rather that you upset yourself by taking your child's misconduct too seriously. At a young age my son stated a common childhood declaration, "I didn't ask to be born!" I replied, "That's right, and if you would have, the answer would have been no!" For one of the few times in his life I had emotionally stopped him in his tracks; he was actually at a loss for words. This little ditty illustrates two important points:

1. With my own brand of humor I had created my own haven, which momentarily stopped my number one son in his tracks— and I thought it couldn't be done! Taking your child's attitudes and behaviors seriously, but yourself lightly, is an important building block.
2. Had I put myself on the defensive, made myself angry about my son's challenge, it would have been highly unlikely that I would have been so creatively light on my feet in my retort. This is where cutting down on your emotional interference has value—it creates clearheadedness first. With a more opened-eyed, lateral-thinking perspective in hand and mind, you can put yourself in a more effective position.

Remember to emotionally lighten up rather than tighten up about your child's sometimes contrary, mischievous behavior. Generating such emotionally insulated havens en route to more visible protective havens can be done by sounding off to yourself the following philosophical examples.

- "Build a haven from your child rather than count on a heaven with her."
- "Pay less heed; indeed, that will be more helpful."
- "I can lighten up preferably while being light on my feet, but also if I fail to say the right thing."
- "I don't have to field my child's curve balls with absolutely no margin for error."
- "Get away and gain a way to recuperate."

- "Slackening up on yourself doesn't mean slackening off as a parent–on the contrary."
- "Douse, don't fan, the flames of your upsets."
- "Be concerned, not consumed."
- "Don't overreact to your child's annoying conduct."
- "Put yourself first and your child a close second."
- "Cool your jets."
- "Chill out."
- "Lighten up."
- "Give yourself permission to be more permissive with yourself."
- "Confront the problem without compounding it."
- "Flow and float through it–don't fight."
- "Fend off, don't feud."

## BEHAVIORAL INSULATION

With your emotions now more in your control rather than at your child's mercy, you can begin to incorporate some of the following protective actions on your own behalf–and as a bonus that you earned from your efforts at emotional self-control–do so in a more effective manner.

a. *Literally get away from it all.* Take a respite when practical by physically distancing yourself for a few days. Such time out can turn out to be a haven on earth by providing emotional relief.

b. *Be a firm communicator.* Tell your child in a no-nonsense manner, "I have no interest in talking to you when you act this way, and I refuse to do so until you stop." Firmly withdraw from the communication exchange to show that you actually mean it.

c. *Find others of like mind.* Attend a parenting class, a parent support group, and find friends and relatives who are looking for their own haven.

d. *Child sharing.* Use the barter system whereby you watch someone else's child in exchange for them watching yours.

e.  *Plan a getaway with a significant other.* Identify places you
    would rather be then minding the store or trying to make your
    child mind. Then brainstorm with one another about re-
    sources you have or how you could get those required to
    follow through with your travels.

f.  *Brainstorm potential places of entertainment and pleasures
    that you can turn to when such an option is practical.* Keep-
    ing such a menu can wet the appetite of hope.

g.  *Plan and scheme with others who relate to your child how to
    manage him in ways that may soften the blows of his difficult
    behavior.* Such a united front against a common enemy pre-
    serves emotional stamina.

h.  *Don't judge yourself.* Whatever you do, don't commit per-
    haps the most anti-mental-health act of all time—self-rating.
    Don't define yourself by your child's behavior so that you
    will be able to more definitely regulate your own emotions.

i.  *Pass the baton.* Give the problem to your child. Do this by
    making the punishment fit the crime while allowing him to
    suffer the natural consequences of his misdeeds. In doing this
    you show him that every decision has a consequence and that
    it is his choice which ones will come his way.

j.  *Seek to master other areas of life.* Get away from constantly
    trying to master the art of parenting. Such repeated efforts on
    the same project can be more than a bit wearing. Seek further
    training for your job that might increase the chances of job
    advancement; passionately take on a special project or special
    interest in line with your natural talents; throw allegiance into
    a special cause you find worthy. All have value in themselves,
    but also and for no extra charge as they provide a safe, produc-
    tive haven from the tussles of parenting.

k.  *Take on a philosophy of benign neglect as a parent.* Float
    through, tune out, blend in with the flow of your child's
    attack rather than meet it head on. Develop the unusual savvy
    of knowing when to just drift away from your problems and
    concerns where you can emotionally and psychologically
    live in a world of your own, as if the real world didn't exist.
    Take a psychological time out when in your best interest to
    do so. With some problems, at times at least, it seems the less

attention paid to them, the less you will experience their emotional wear and tear–and the sooner they will either go away or be experienced less harshly.

Children and adolescents frequently make themselves dependent on being independent of their parents. Such ambitions carry with them a fair amount of intrusive, oppositional activities. Use the two-phased approach described in this chapter, inner control and outer protection, to take a tough-minded rather than a tough-knuckled approach toward parenting. This will put you in a better position to fend off rather than feud with your offspring. Such civilized deflections and diffusions may not pave the way to heaven on earth. However, just as the road to hell is paved with good intentions, so too will good intentions–backed by the right protective methods–provide you with an earthly haven from which to comfort and rejuvenate yourself.

# Chapter 29

# The Only Golden Rule
# of Parenting

Parents are besieged with recipes for successful parenting. Do this, i.e., hug your child at least X number of times per day; do that, i.e., be consistent in your management of him; do the other thing, i.e., be a day-in and day-out if not a minute-by-minute positive role model for your supposed imitative child. It seems that all the child requires to be emotionally healthy is perfect parents who follow somebody else's prescriptions for success. In part because it is easier to be a hero to someone else's problems, parents are often advised as to what they "should," "must," "have to," "ought to," are "supposed to" do as parents. It is the contention of this chapter that this absolute dogma produces problems rather than remedies, and that it would be emotionally healthier to adopt the position that "the only golden rule of parenting is: There is no golden rule."

As a consequence of relying on golden-rule certainty, parents put undo pressure on themselves, heighten expectations to an unrealistic level only to discover that once reality kills the golden rule, the emotional fallout is that much greater. By following all the absolute rules and regulations, parents miss out on much of the potential joy and opportunity in their parenting responsibilities. Although there are guidelines for doing justice to the parenting role, the split second such preferential suggestions are elevated into perfectionistic demands (or golden rules) a decent respect for individual differences as well as a harnessing of emotional well-being is lost. There are many disadvantages of righteously holding up absolute standards to be applied without fail. Such insistences hasten turning the solution into the problem. A smattering of such "necessities" as fed to and/or created by parents are:

- "I absolutely must have open communication with my child."
- "I need to find solutions to any and all of my child's problems and concerns."
- "It is necessary that I provide a standard of living that is at least on par, if not slightly or more above his peers."
- "I should never yell at my child."
- "I must never lay a finger on my child."
- "I have to get my child to responsibly follow society's rules."
- "I'm supposed to get my child to at least be a bit interested in school."
- "It is up to me and therefore I should find constructive ways for my child to structure her time."
- "I must see to it that my child doesn't use drugs or be a part of a teenage pregnancy."
- "I have to gain my child's understanding and acceptance of house rules and a moral compliance and agreement on what's right and what's wrong."
- "I must always provide my child with a steady role model."
- "I must never show weakness, or admit fault and error to my child; If I am a man I should never cry in front of my child–especially a son."

The list of what parents are "supposed" to be doing as parents and how they are "supposed" to do it goes on, but it is sufficient to say that presumed royalty, if not sacred notions, have the net effect of creating the following disadvantages:

1. *Lock yourself into an emotional double bind.* Doing something because some arbitrary authority says that you "should" encourages resentment toward such dictates, while going against what those folks declare you "should" do–cultivates guilt and a "damned if you do, damned if you don't" arrangement.

2. *Causes pent-up emotions.* As soon as you tell yourself as a parent that you "have to" do a certain thing, you will feel an immediate cringing in the pit of your gut. This is a signal that your white-knuckled approach to parent-child issues has you emotionally cooked.

3. *Creates an emotional roller coaster.* As long as you follow

golden rule declarations you may find some emotional comfort. However, because it is unlikely that you will succeed at never failing, when you do flounder you will likely bottom yourself out emotionally.

4. *Causes tunnel vision.* A restricted view follows the belief that there are definite paths to parenting that I "must" follow.

5. *Detracts from free will while discouraging you from thinking for yourself.* Buying into almighty, "holier than thou" pronouncements as to how you "ought to" conduct yourself as a parent disparages your own abilities to think for yourself. Instead of marching to the beat of your own drummer, you practice the bad habit of stepping to the sound of someone elses'.

6. *Chills individual difference.* What might be good for some, or even most, concerning child management, may not fit for you. Often, selecting solutions to parenting problems that don't go by the book may make you glad that you didn't read the book.

7. *Blocks alternatives.* "The way" of doing things doesn't leave room for other, more well-rounded possibilities.

8. *Increases stress and tension.* Pressure is fueled by trying to find something that doesn't exist—the absolute truths of the "got to's."

9. *Detracts from hope.* When the golden rules don't get you out of the starting blocks, hopes are dashed due to the limited alternatives that make up "the way" to parent.

10. *Abolishes creative parenting.* Optional thinking is much more likely to occur in a climate of permissiveness, with fewer limitations of thought, rather than in an undemocratic one.

11. *Ensures self-blame, blocks (undamning) self-acceptance.* Violation of the universal standards at the core of the "have to's" and "shoulds" will likely lead to self-downing.

12. *Betrays the reality of human limitations.* Humans cannot succeed at each and every outing. However, dogmatic ways of thinking do not allow for such possibilities.

13. *Disallows the human right to be wrong.* A "must" or one of the other similar black-or-white, all-or-nothing parental phi-

losophies implies that each and every time, under all conditions, the individual "must" act in a certain manner. This rigid idea runs counter to ordinary human inconsistency.

14. *Is often followed by discomfort despisement.* The insistent "should" brings on the pressure and frustration, which is frequently followed by aggravation and overreaction to the stress itself. Exaggerating the significance of discomfort will only cause it to pyramid further.

15. *Seeks perfectionism and the gateway to heaven.* Looking for things that don't exist creates a problem that has a life of its own. The above two pie-in-the-sky searchings are better off destroyed if happiness is to be salvaged.

The implications that lie behind the "have to's" are that if I don't do what I "should" do as a parent:

- "It's terrible, horrendous, and catastrophic."
- "I can't stand it or myself because I didn't do what was allegedly required."
- "I'm a bad person for following my own lead rather than someone elses' mandates."

These ideas can be challenged by such statements/questions as:

- "It's not a question of what should I do, but what do I really want to do about this circumstance involving my child?"
- "Who would know more about what I think is best in this matter with my child—a theorist writing about the topic, or a realist like myself living it out?"
- "I thought this was a democratic state, not a fascist one where the leaders define absolutistic ideas to live by."
- "One size doesn't fit all and likely never did or will. Now what decision fits for this child, at this time?"
- "I'm not going to set myself up for disappointment by pretending that there is only one way to going about managing a parent-child problem."
- "It's the same old story: There is no (absolute) way for me to transplant a different attitude into my child's head, nor a different feeling into his gut."

- "Let me use my free will to decide, not allow some dictator to dictate."
- "Let me brainstorm how many different ways there are to look at this problem rather than presume there is only one."
- "Universal laws imply arrogance and self-righteousness and there is already enough of that in the world."
- "If the 'should' rule doesn't work out, where does that leave me as far as hope goes? Better that I leave my options open."
- "I have a right to be wrong, to try and fail—my way."
- "Following someone else's rules to the letter of the law only encourages resentment on my part."

Such self-statements allow for more latitude, permissiveness, open-mindedness, and flexibility resulting in discouraging the establishment of sacred standards that limit decision-making alternatives. Be aware of prescriptions that lock you into one mode of parenting that provides some security and comfort in the short run, but leaves you with emotional fallout in the long run. Test out guidelines that seem to hold some sensible logic in your approach to parenting. However, avoid dogmatic recipes for parenting methods. Until evidence to the contrary presents itself, always remember that there are no golden rules of parenting.

Chapter 30

# Wiles of My Own Parenting
# to Date

Writing a book about imperfect parents, of imperfect children, in an imperfect family is many times easier than being an imperfect parent, of imperfect children, in an imperfect family. I am writing this chapter at the risk of making a common human mistake of overgeneralizing, i.e., implying that this is what it (parenting) was like for me and because my size fits all, let me tell you what is right for you. This is akin to a family member's declaration, "If I want your opinion, I'll give it to you." Parents sometimes inquire of me in their own direct and/or indirect manner, "OK, Bub, since you know so much about solving family problems, what goofs did you make as a parent–and what blunders are you continuing to make?" Being the active-directive therapist that I usually am, I will frequently respond, "Are you sure you have the time–and the stomach–for it all?" Such a transparent response (a) models my fallibility as a human-parent, (b) signals the client that, "Yes, you heard me correctly–I'm one of you," and (c) demonstrates to the parent that because the matter of parenting does matter, it doesn't have to be taken as seriously as it oftentimes is. That the parent can care less without becoming uncaring.

I was asked on a radio talk show, "What do you think is the biggest sin, or error of omission, that a parent can commit?" Good question, I thought. After a brief hesitation I gave what I thought was a reasonably good answer: "I think the biggest mistake that a parent can commit is to hold themselves accountable for the *inevitable* problems that their children will have." In spite of my own errors of parenting, I aim for "undamning acceptance" of myself, in spite of parental flaws and deficiencies. I think that until we as parents can learn to accept ourselves with our shortcomings (present company included) we will be too upset about our mistakes to correct them. Alfred Adler said, "It's easier to fight for your ideals than to live up to them." Accepting yourself with your blunders is an ideal similar to shooting for the bulls eye in archery. You're not going to hit it every time, but because you have a bead on it, you're likely to hit it or come closer to it more often.

Do the child rearing and family therapist experts have fewer personal, parenting, or family problems? I doubt it. Mark Twain said, "To be good is noble, to teach others to be good is more noble yet–and less of a hassle." Most humans–counselors and noncounselors alike-choose to avoid the extra hassle because it is the most convenient thing to do. Good advice is much easier to give than it is to follow. That doesn't mean it's not good advice–just that it's easier to provide than apply; knowledge is light years apart from action/application. There is the story of an expert on parent-child relationships who wrote a book called *Ten **Rules** for Raising Children.* After his first child he wrote another text, *Ten **Suggestions** for Raising Children,* and after his second child he wrote *Ten **Hints** for Raising Children.* After his third child he wrote no more books. Another family therapy expert was overheard saying, "Before I had kids I had four theories about bringing up children and now I have four kids–and no theories about child rearing!"

This expert has raised two children who defy the odds of the laws of learning, role modeling, and the impact of family values, and who reflected the idea that the trouble with child psychology is that children don't understand it. Both were raised under the same roof, exposed to consistently similar values, but yet are a picture of contrasts. My son would rather hunt and fish than eat. My daughter is a dyed-in-the-wool vegetarian, is highly selective in what she eats, and is an animal rights activist to boot. My daughter was an excellent student, my son "academically disinclined"; I learned more than I ever cared to learn at his parent-teacher conferences that I faithfully attended. My son was a communicator par excellence–he would literally run into the house eagerly wanting to tell my wife and I about his day; my daughter would tell us very little about her time away from home. My son is highly sociable and keeps more friendly acquaintances than you can shake a stick at; my daughter is quite selective in who she will pal around with. The differences almost too numerous to mention continue to go on. Don't tell me something's not up that goes well beyond the conventional ideas that children learn what they see, and therefore, mirror family happenings and values. I support the theory that children develop more by nature than nurture. They inherit temperamental and value tendencies, exhibit these tendencies in their family, and will do this apart from whatever goes or doesn't go on in their family of origin. Children will simply follow their own direction and usually a team of wild horses can't keep their nature in check—to say nothing about bringing their tendencies to a screeching halt. Children will simply continue to express their tendencies, which in some cases will be for better and in other cases for worse. These inclinations are powerful, but not binding. In the case of the "for worse," tendencies can be controlled or made not to be binding. Such a transformation practically always occurs after a jolt from a life experience that results in a heavy consequence for expression of these tendencies. At that point the person may decide to keep such expressions down to a roar—run them before they ruin him. Anna Freud said that life is the best possible teacher. After a series of negative results, with severe consequences for bad decisions, the individual may decide to make better decisions that lead to better consequences, having learned that every decision has a consequence. After life provides a rude awakening, the child may decide to bring his or her self-defeating tendencies—e.g., a build-up and/or expression of anger; education deficiencies; excesses in food, alcohol, nicotine; procrastinating oneself out of house and home; fickleness in bonding relationships; neglect of general health; employment instability—under better control. Until these circumstances impact on the child, the parent is afforded the luxury of using the wiles of his or her parenting role to work on his or her own emotional stability.

Back to yours truly. In short, my daughter with all her quietude was a low-maintenance child, while my son with all his expression was a high-maintenance child; she was an experience, he an adventure. Stories and stormy anecdotes from my adventures in my son's upbringing include:

- His second grade teacher conference told of an art class assignment in which the class was asked to draw a turtle. Everyone completed the assignment except Billy who had scribbled all over his paper. The teacher checked out all the turtles until she came to Billy's scribbling and asked him, "Billy, I thought that I told you to draw a turtle. How come you didn't draw one?" To which Billy stated, "I *did* draw a turtle: The turtle is in the muck." Apparently there is more than one way to look at things.
- On a rainy Sunday afternoon when he was about five years old he began shooting his popgun (because I believe in training them young). Unfortunately, his mother was taking a nap at the same time so I instructed him, "Billy, would you knock off shooting your popgun? Your mother's taking a nap." He responded, "What do you expect me to do?" I countered, "Just make believe you're shooting your popgun." After a pause he replied, "I've got a better idea, Dad. Why don't you just tell Mom to make believe she's sleeping." At about that point I was ready to call my social worker (but they don't work on weekends).
- When he was about age seven I instructed him to put his clothes in the wash right side out; he quickly shot back, "Well, what do you know—my Dad turned into a Mom." Then they wonder why I believe that if I can make my children miserable one more time, I'll be convinced that I have done my job.
- At about age six after Billy had made a mess of the basement, I foolishly proceeded to chew him out. He gave me the time of day to hear me out, after which he surveyed the damage and noticed, among all his debris, one of my socks. After focusing on that sock to a point of practically staring a hole through it, he looked up at me and with a twinkle in his eye retorted, "Nice try, Dad." Right then and there I began to wonder where I went wrong.
- Around age ten he and his sister Barb were arguing about who was going to wash and who was going to wipe the dishes. I burst into their arguing and forcefully stated, "Decide who is going to wash and who is going to wipe—or go to your rooms."

Billy calmly looked at Barb and inquired, "What should we do, Barb?" Obviously children have gotten harder to scare.

- We were opening our Christmas presents when my son was six. Billy noticed that his sister, who is a year older than he, got a camera but he didn't. He began acting rather obnoxiously so I said, "Billy, what the heck is the problem?" He spritely shot back, "Man, can't a guy be a little jealous?" Some kids will swear by your rewards and some will swear at them.
- Around age eight one of Billy's baby teeth fell out. (No, I didn't knock it out.) As he kissed me goodnight that evening he handed me an envelope and scooted off to bed. Glancing at the envelope it read, "To the Tooth Fairy–$2 minimum."
- At about age seven after correcting a piece of his behavior, he didn't appreciate my doing so. He began to boisterously challenge me, at which point I directed him to go to his room. As he slowly but surely moved toward his room he loudly protested my direct order to get to his room. I had read someplace that bad behavior gone unnoticed will eventually extinguish itself. Thus, I ignored him. He finally got to his room and began to realize it was going to be difficult for him to get under my skin. Not to be denied, there was a long pause from his end and I sensed he was going to come forth with a last-ditch effort to get me to overreact to his discontent. He finally replied, "And one more thing, Dad. I'm not your buddy anymore, either." Emotional disturbance is handed down; children hand it down to their parents. But what's a house without children? Answer: (a) quiet, (b) paid for. Get the picture?

I would like to further explain my relationship and status with my two children, now both young adults. I consider my number one achievement as a parent to be that through all our differences and different ways of going through life, my son and I remain openly and unashamedly fond of one another, still hugging with a kiss and an "I love you" after a visit. The biggest mistake I made as a parent was to presume the sacredness of the role itself, believing it to be the most important, creative thing one can do in a lifetime. In preparation for my parenting role, I studied the topic like I had not studied any topic before or since the onset of my offspring. In my attempts to carry out what I studied I reserved huge amounts of time to be with my children, wrongly believing that a relationship with parents is the primary molder of a child's personality. How wrong I was! But live and learn. Most can become a parent, but it takes a wise person to know when to get off the parental train. Before you get off the train you have a moral obligation to try to do well as a parent. Once you have done that, get off the train and get on with the rest of your life. I gave myself (and to some degree still do) some difficulty in backing away from and getting off the parental train. This was due to my perspective of the task; I saw it as the ultimate importance, rather than simply important.

I truly have learned the value of a decent respect for individual differences through my day-to-day experiences with my children—much more so than through any other context. My daughter, who naturally shares and patronizes my values, and I got along with a minimum of conflict in the child-rearing years. My son Bill, who openly talked back to my values, and I didn't get along as well during those younger years. However, I believe that you learn more from someone who doesn't think like you—though there may be more conflictual sparks in the process. Consequently, although Barb and I were much more alike and compatible, I can honestly say that I learned much more from my son. The moral of this last story is that I remain eternally grateful to both my children—in different ways.

# Index

Page numbers followed by the letter "t" indicate tables; those followed by the letter "f" indicate figures.